Filler Complications

Ik Soo Koh · Won Lee

Filler Complications

Filler-Induced Hypersensitivity Reactions, Granuloma, Necrosis, and Blindness

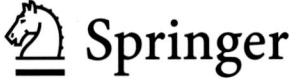 Springer

Ik Soo Koh
KohIkSoo Plastic Surgery Clinic
Seoul
South Korea

Won Lee
Yonsei E1 Plastic Surgery Clinic
Anyang
Kyonggi-do
South Korea

ISBN 978-981-13-6638-3   ISBN 978-981-13-6639-0   (eBook)
https://doi.org/10.1007/978-981-13-6639-0

Library of Congress Control Number: 2019935526

This Springer imprint is published by the registered company Springer Nature Singapore Pte Ltd. The registered company address is: 152 Beach Road, #21-01/04 Gateway East, Singapore 189721, Singapore

Preface

Filler injection is a commonly performed cosmetic procedure that has greatly progressed in the last decade. However, there remains a lack of evidence-based knowledge and scientific experience. My goal for this book was to share my experience with filler complications and provide precise injection guidance to prevent filler complications.

For this first English edition, I worked carefully to organize my knowledge of filler complications based on my experience with the 2015 Korean edition of the book. Writing a book is hard work, so I am thankful that I was able to persevere and publish this book with tremendous effort.

I also wish to thank to my family, colleagues, and especially my mother, Hwa-Ja Lee, with respect and love.

Ik-Soo Koh
President of APAS
Director of KohIkSoo Plastic Surgery Clinic
Seoul, South Korea

Although I am a plastic surgeon, patients now frequently request that I perform more minor procedures, such as botulinum toxin injections, filler injections, and thread lifting, because their desires have changed over the last decade. Therefore, I needed to study about fillers. This book provides the proper answers to questions about filler rheology, injection guidance, anatomy, and filler complications. It was a great honor to publish this book, which contains the tremendous experience of Dr. Koh.

As always, I give thanks to SeungHyun, HyunJi, and JounYoun with love.

Won Lee
Director of Yonsei E1 Plastic Surgery Clinic
Kyonggi-do, South Korea

Recommendations

"Dr. Koh always insists on using the correct procedures, while Dr. Lee is always trying to solve problems for the audience during speeches. I greatly respect these two great surgeons." Wook Oh, MD, President of KALDAT, South Korea

"Reading this book will make your injections perfect!" JinLiang Lee, MD, Justmake Plastic Surgery Clinic, Taipei, Taiwan

"As the specialty of aesthetic medicine evolves, books like this are valuable contributions to such a highly specialized field. This essential book helps to give patients a safe and enjoyable experience by providing a deep understanding of what can go wrong. That's why this book is a great reference for any aesthetic physician." Jani A.J. van Loghem, MD, Amsterdam, The Netherlands

"Drs. Koh and Lee explain a variety of granulomatous formations and vascular complications from fillers in an easy-to-understand format. I personally recommend that all injectors read this book to treat their patients with safe and effective techniques." Rungsima Wanitphakdeedecha, MD, Bangkok, Thailand

"How can we find a perfect balance in this imperfect science? It is not just medical knowledge—it is an art! Dr. Lee is not just a plastic surgeon; he is also an inventor and an artist!" Ben-li Chan, MD, Style Aesthetics Clinic, Taichung, Taiwan

Contents

About the Authors

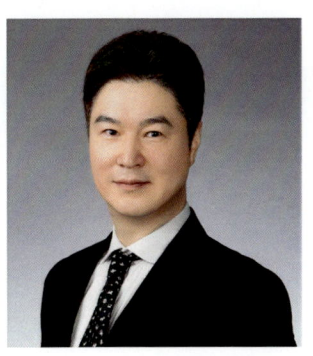

Ik-Soo Koh is a plastic surgeon. He received his M.D. and Ph.D. from College of Medicine, Hanyang University, Seoul, South Korea. Currently, he is the Director of KohIkSoo Plastic Surgery Clinic.

Dr. Koh has worldwide reputation as an authority in the field of filler injections. He was the faculty of IMCAS, Asia, and the president of international symposium of minimal invasive plastic surgery in Bangkok and Shanghai. He was the president of the Minimal invasive Plastic Surgery of Korean Society of Plastic and Reconstructive Surgeons. Currently, Dr. Koh is the president of the Association of Petit Aesthetic Surgery (APAS) and still dedicating to share his tremendous experience of filler injection and filler complications.

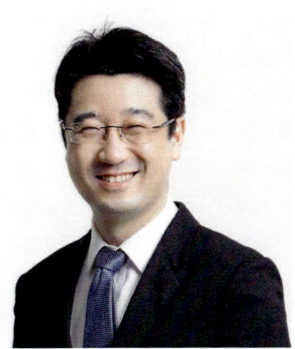

Won Lee is a plastic surgeon. He received his M.D. from Yonsei University Medical College and Ph. D. from College of Medicine, Dongguk University, Seoul, South Korea. Currently, he is the Director of Yonsei E1 Plastic Surgery Clinic, Anyang.

Dr. Lee is the member of the Korean Society of Plastic and Reconstructive Surgeons and member of the Minimal invasive Plastic Surgery, South Korea. He wrote various papers about the filler, which are "Practical guidelines for hyaluronic acid soft tissue filler use in facial rejuvenation (*Dermatologic Surgery*)," "Effective of retrobulbar hyaluronidase injection in an iatrogenic blindness rabbit model using hyaluronic acid filler injections (*Plastic and Reconstructive Surgery*)," and "Novel technique of filler injection in the temple area (*Journal of Plastic, Reconstructive and Aesthetic Surgeons*)" and still investigating various experiments about filler injection and filler complications.

Classification of Filler Complications

A "petit procedure" is a minor procedure such as an injection that immediately changes the face. Soft-tissue filler injections are among the most widely used petit procedures to improve scars and wrinkles and provide soft-tissue augmentation. Such procedures are quite simple for patients and doctors. However, anatomical knowledge and an understanding of the filler's properties are required because the procedure is performed blindly. It is why doctor feels more and more difficult when doing more procedure.

Patient quality of life could increase if the filler injection result is highly satisfactory, but it could decrease if the result is unsatisfactory or complications occur. Filler injections are safe procedures compared to other plastic procedures, but complications can cause stress for both patients and doctors. Accordingly, it is very important that doctors be knowledgeable about potential filler complications and patients be aware of minimal complications like bruising or swelling. This chapter will introduce generalized and organized classification information about filler complications to help ensure safe filler injection technique.

1.1 Etiology and Classification of Patient Dissatisfaction

Filler injection is an essential procedure in the aesthetic medical field. According to the American Society of Plastic Surgeons, an estimated 2.7 million procedures were performed at 2017.

The usage of filler has increased tremendously. Some cases of rhinoplasty are being replaced by filler injection. However, filler complications are also increasing due to its increased use. Most of all, clinicians must be aware of possible severe problems like skin necrosis and blindness, the incidence of which is also increasing.

We can classify patient dissatisfaction as follows (Table 1.1).

We can classify the causes of these complaints as follows:

– Medical malpractice.
– Patient did not follow care instructions.
– Filler's unique property.
– Patient's subjective view.

It is difficult to attribute an unsatisfactory result to one specific cause since it is usually

Table 1.1 Patient dissatisfactions

Point of view	Irregular shape
	Looks spread and wide
	Noticeable through the skin
	Located in places other than the injection site
Physical feel	Hard
	Touchable
	Unable to touch
	Able to touch other site
Subjective assessment	Blunt
	Thin
	Weird
	Unflattering

© Springer Nature Singapore Pte Ltd. 2019
I. S. Koh, W. Lee, *Filler Complications*, https://doi.org/10.1007/978-981-13-6639-0_1

due to a combination of two or three causes. For example, irregularity occurs due to medical malpractice, but it could also be a result of the filler's easy spreading property or a patient's wrongdoing such as pressing on the area. Thus, it is important to photograph the area before and immediately after the filler injection.

1.2   Classification of Complications

Filler complication follows a traditional process because it has definite cause. The most important factor is onset time, which can provide many clues for proper treatment (Table 1.2).

1.3   Bruising and Swelling

Bruising is the most common minor complication. Bruises change color from red wine to red to yellow step by step. Severe bruising can involve many different colors. Vessel rupture and blood stagnation are the causes of bruising. Bruising is sometimes seen below the injection site because blood is moving downward through the subcutaneous layer by gravity.

Swelling usually peaks 24–48 hours after the injection and then subsides. It is important to warn patients that swelling will worsen but should not be cause for alarm. Besides these natural processes, if extensive subcutaneous hemorrhage occurs, swelling with hardness may develop. Calcium hydroxyapatite filler or polycaprolactone filler tends to cause immediate swelling and likely prolonged swelling for 2 hours, so it is important to know the natural course of the swelling process.

Hyaluronic acid filler also shows differences in swelling due to differences in chemical con-

Table 1.2 Complication classified by onset time

Immediate after injection	Bruising, swelling, erythema, blindness
Early (1 day to 1 week)	Swelling, erythema, infection, dermatitis, allergy, skin necrosis
Late (1 week or later)	Pigmentation, migration, filler induced hypersensitivity reaction granuloma

Table 1.3 Causes of swelling by time

Immediate after injection	Subcutaneous hemorrhage
2–4 hours	Unique properties of products like calcium hydroxyapatite filler or polycaprolactone filler
24–48 hours	Normal progress
>48 hours	Aggravating swelling and pain suggest infection
1 week	Delayed swelling

centrations and manufacturing processes. This will be described in more detail in Chap. 2.

When swelling is prolonged (>48 hours), patients should be told to seek medical help for possible infection (Table 1.3).

1.3.1   Treatment

There are several methods for reducing bruising and swelling. Ointments containing vitamin K or light-emitting diode (LED) phototherapy may be advisable. Ice compression might be done at the clinic but is not advisable at the patient's home because the filler might be excessively compressed.

1.3.2   Prevention

The most common site of bruising is the puncture site. To reduce the risk of bruising, the linear threading technique has advantages over the serial puncture technique. Basically, the use of fewer puncture sites carries a lower chance of bruising.

After puncturing, needle movement should be minimal to avoid tissue or vessel damage. The needle tip should be advanced gently through the avascular layer. For example, when injecting filler into the nose, it is relatively safe to inject it into the supraperiosteal layer because it has fewer vessels than the other layers. It is extremely important to know which layers are relatively safe and which are major vessel pathways. It is better to make the injection under bright light because some female patients' skin is thin enough for the practitioner to detect small vessels.

1.4 Erythema

Temporary erythema during the 10 minutes after the injection is a normal human reaction. However, erythema that persists for >24 hours indicates a circulation disturbance caused by filler compression of the vessel and disturbances in blood influx and outflux. Compression pressure decreases, and erythema can be diminished by stretching of the skin at the filler injection site. Thus, we can define erythema as minor vessel compression. Increased compression pressure could lead to skin necrosis, so we must carefully observe patient progress when erythema appears.

1.4.1 Etiology

Erythema occurs in areas of little skin redundancy. For example, when filler is injected into the dorsum of the nose, the pressure spreads to the adjacent tissues; in contrast, when it is injected into the tip of the nose, it is in a solitary area subjected to all of the pressure and tends to show erythema.

A previous scar can change vascular microcirculation, while a previous implant can create a capsule surrounding the implant. Either of these situations may disturb the circulation and lead to erythema (Figs. 1.1 and 1.2).

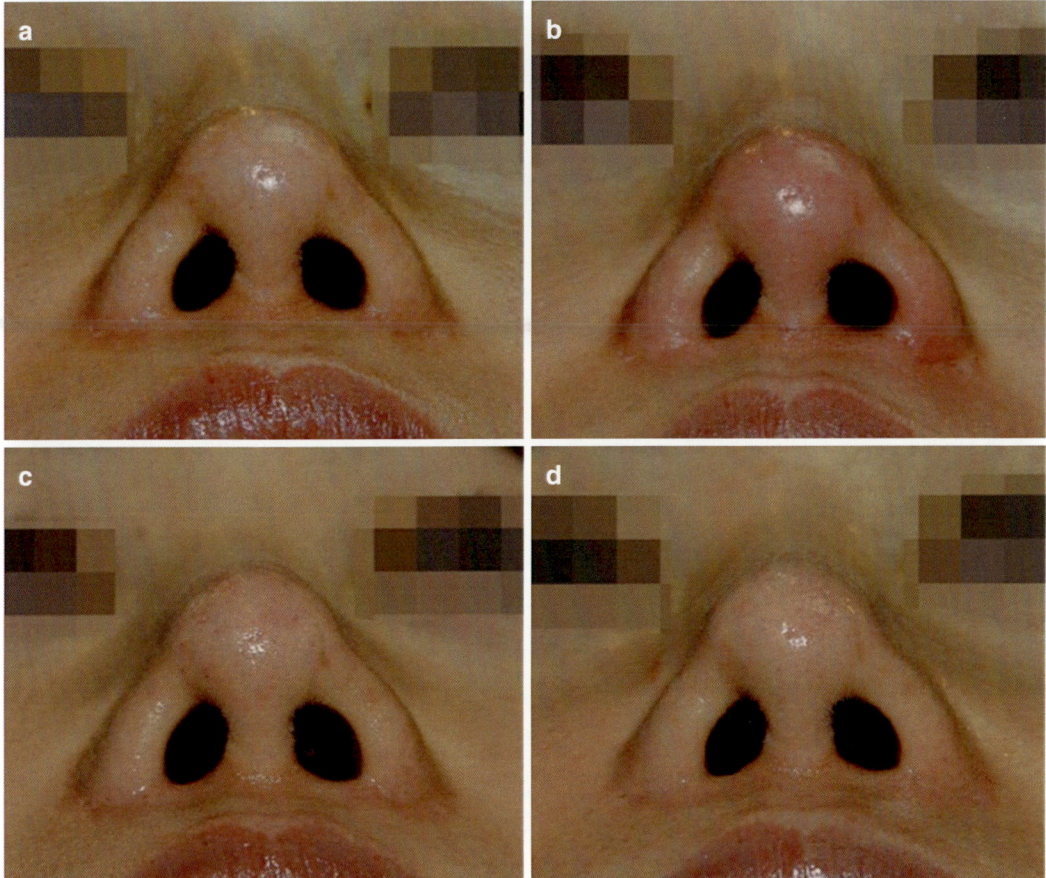

Fig. 1.1 Erythema of previous open rhinoplasty patient, self-healed. Previous open rhinoplasty and alar reduction patient. Hyaluronic acid filler 0.2cc was injected and erythema persisted for 2 weeks and self healed in 2 months. Erythema develops easily after previous rhinoplasty due to changes in the vasculature. (**a**) Preoperative view. (**b**) Erythema immediately after the injection. (**c**) 2 weeks after injection, localized erythema persisted. (**d**) Two months after the injection, the erythema disappeared

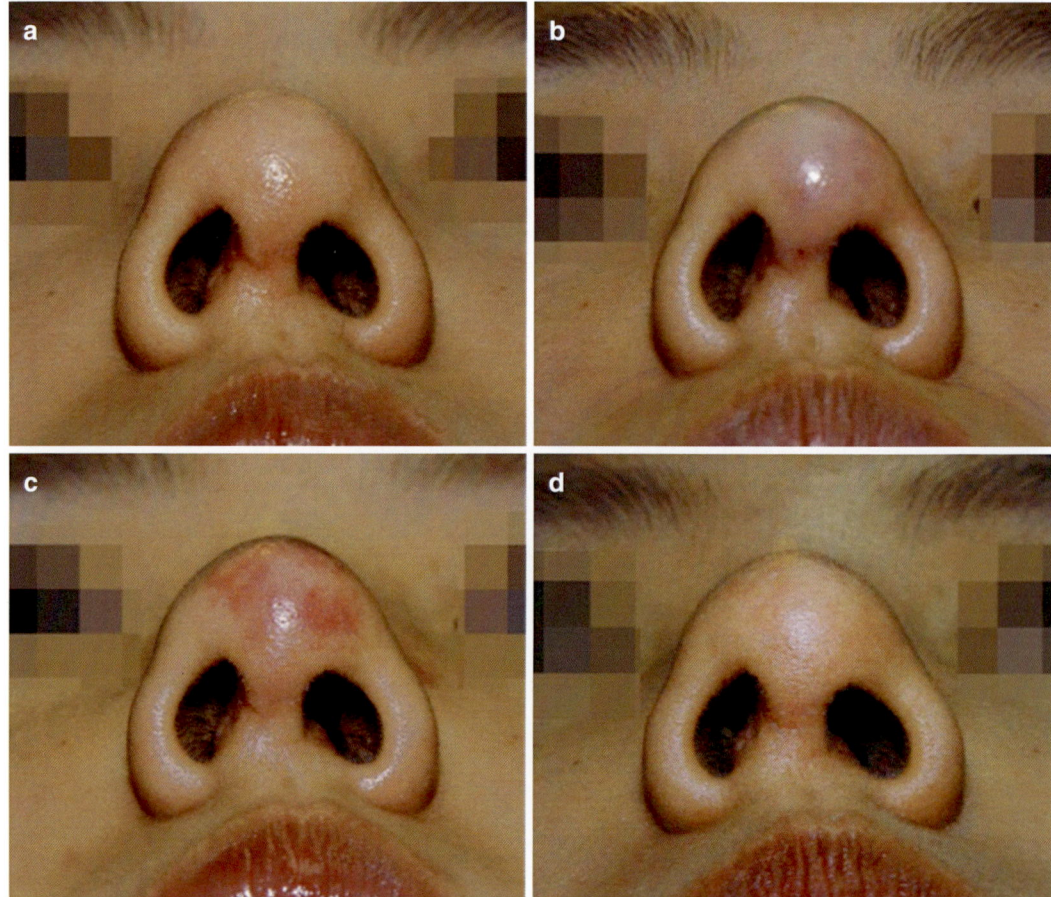

Fig. 1.2 Erythema of previous multiple open rhinoplasty patient. Hyaluronidase induced healing. Severe scar tissue due to previous multiple open rhinoplasty. Hyaluronic acid filler 0.1 cc was injected into the nasal tip, which was immediately blanched. Three days after the erythema developed, the area was healed by injected hyaluronidase. (**a**) Preoperative view. (**b**) Immediate after the injection. (**c**) Three days after the injection, the erythema developed. (**d**) Three weeks after the injection, the erythema disappeared

Some semipermanent fillers, such as polymethylmethacrylate (PMMA) or calcium hydroxyapatite filler, tend to create a separate layer and could disturb the circulation, so secondary procedures with this kind of filler should be performed carefully (Fig. 1.3).

1.4.2 Treatment

The basic procedure involves decompression. Since erythema is caused by a circulation disturbance induced by compression pressure, decompression as soon as possible is the key to preventing skin necrosis. Aggressive decompression is indicated when the following occur:

- Immediate blanching
- Progressive erythema 10 minutes after the injection
- Excessive tension feeling at the injection site
- Progressive erythema and pain 2 days after the injection

Decompression methods differ by filler properties.

Fig. 1.3 Erythema of previous PMMA filler injection. A patient who previously underwent PMMA filler injection experienced erythema at the previous injection site after polyacrylamide gel filler injection that self-healed after 3 months. (**a**) Preoperative view. (**b**) Ten days after the injection. (**c**) Fourteen days after the injection. (**d**) Three months after the injection

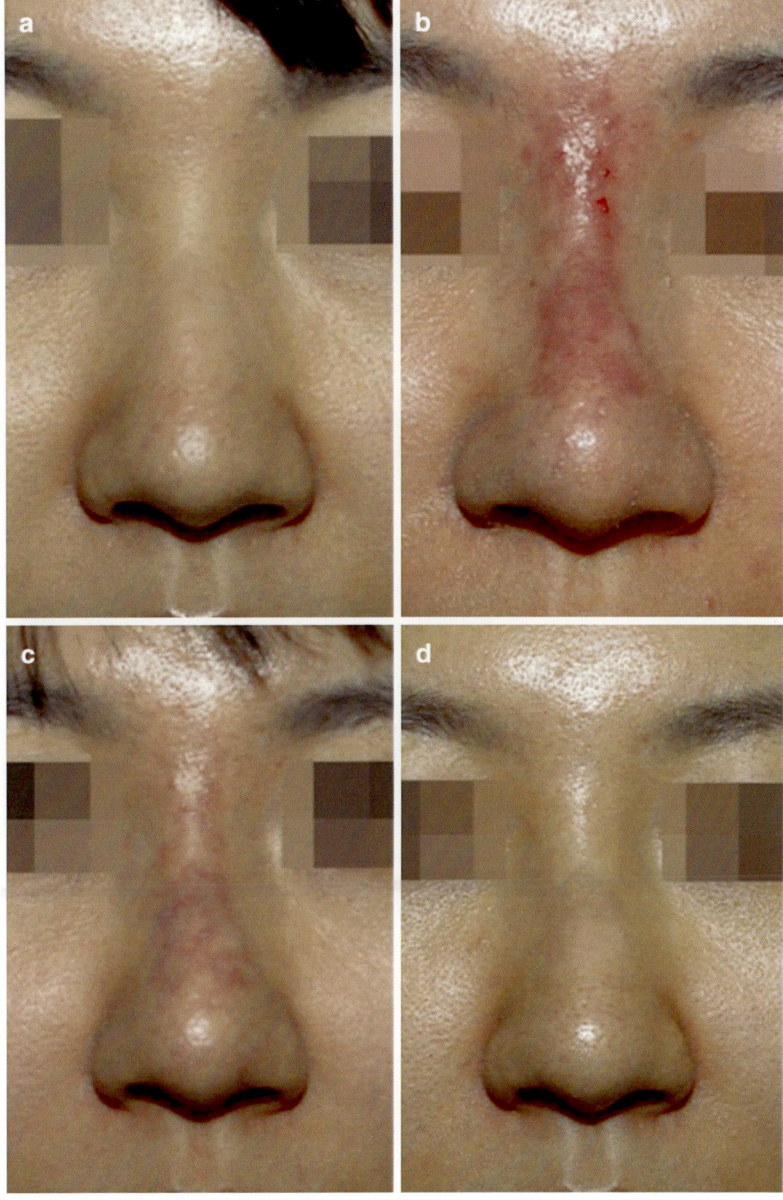

Hyaluronidase is injected in cases of hyaluronic acid filler. When the decision is made to dissolve the filler, the use of a sufficient amount of substrate is appropriate. Saving some of the filler inside the skin to maintain the shape cannot stop the progression to skin necrosis. Rather, all filler should be dissolved, the skin left to stabilize, and the filler reinjected. Mixing 1–1.5 cc of normal saline into one vial of hyaluronidase powder (1500 IU) prevents introducing more pressure during the injection of hyaluronidase.

PMMA or polyacrylamide gel filler should be removed using 18G needle aspiration with negative pressure (Fig. 1.4).

Calcium hydroxyapatite filler remains in a liquid state until 2 weeks. As the gel carriers are absorbed, fillers become more solid. This is the

なし

why fillers can be removed by aspiration before 2 weeks (Figs. 1.5, 1.6, and 1.7).

The PMMA filler may be removable by aspiration 1–2 weeks after injection; thereafter, surgery is required. It forms very hard particles called artificial bone and aggregates with normal tissue, making it very difficult to remove.

The collagen filler also transforms to solid particles 1–2 days after injection; thereafter, it is also difficult to remove by aspiration (Fig. 1.8).

After decompression, the use of antibiotics and anti-inflammatory drugs to prevent more severe ischemic damage should be considered. In cases of minor ischemic damage, erythema subsides immediately after decompression, but when ischemic damage is severe, de-epithelization or a skin infection might occur after decompression.

1.5 Infection

There are several causes of infection (Table 1.4).

Injection syringe or needle contamination is rare. If the injection kit is contaminated, the filler is also contaminated, and a soft-tissue infection is introduced when the needle passes through the skin multiple times. To prevent this

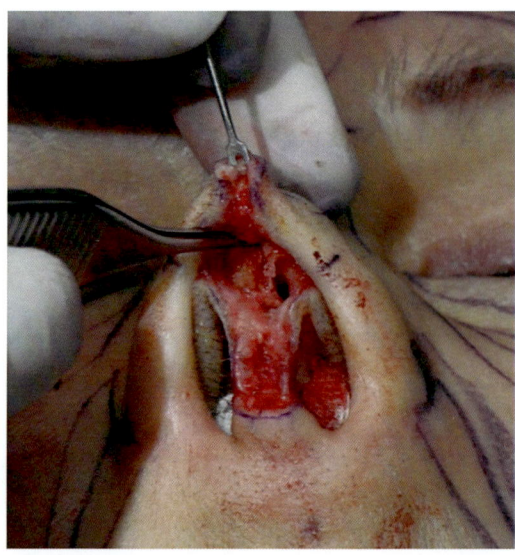

Fig. 1.6 Removal of calcium hydroxyapatite filler (after 2 weeks). Two weeks after injection, calcium hydroxyapatite filler tends to change to a solid product that cannot be removed by needle aspiration. In such cases, surgery is required. Calcium hydroxyapatite filler transformed to solid material 3 months after injection

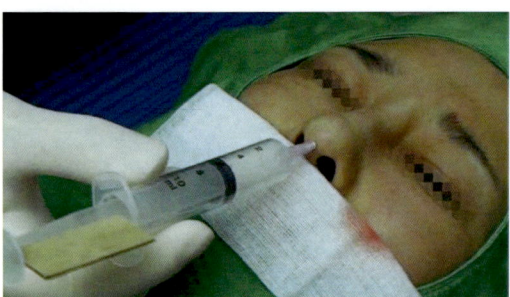

Fig. 1.4 Removal of polyacrylamide gel filler. Needle aspiration using negative pressure. Nose augmentation with polyacrylamide gel filler 7 years prior

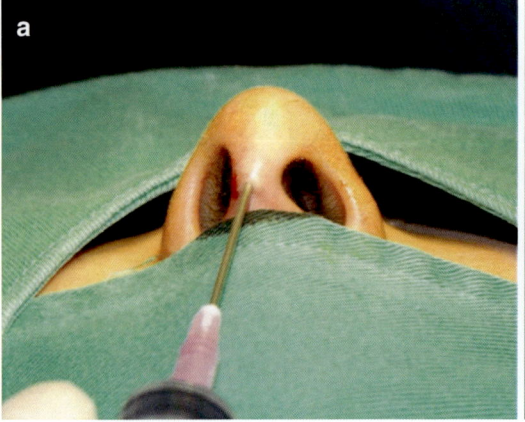
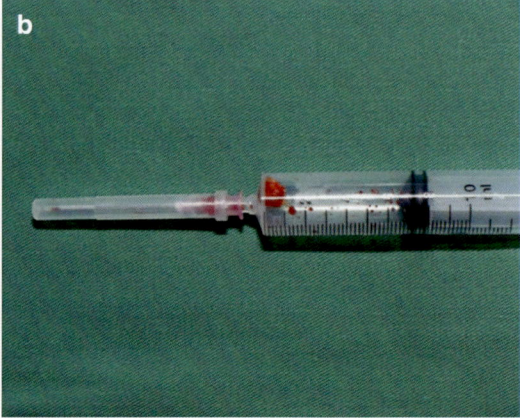

Fig. 1.5 Removal of calcium hydroxyapatite filler (before 2 weeks). (**a**) Removal of calcium hydroxyapatite filler using 18G negative pressure aspiration. (**b**) Removed calcium hydroxyapatite filler in syringe

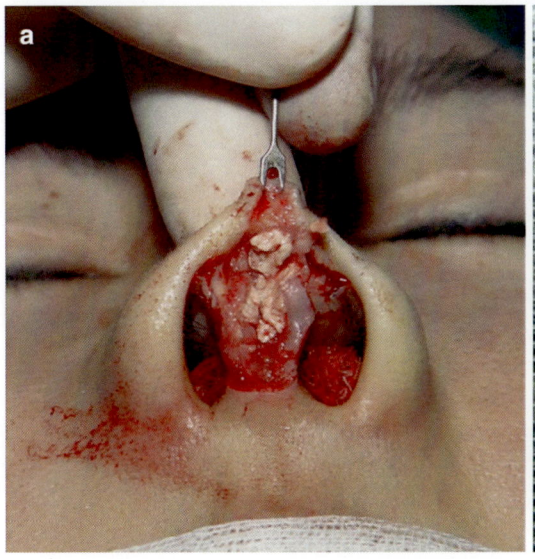
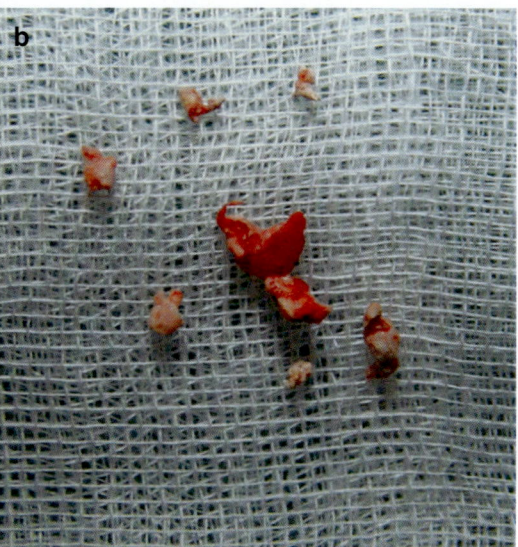

Fig. 1.7 Removal of calcium hydroxyapatite filler (after 2 weeks). Operative view: calcium hydroxyapatite filler findings during open rhinoplasty. (**a**) Calcium particles having aggregated with the adjacent tissue 6 months after the injection. (**b**) Removed calcium hydroxyapatite filler particles

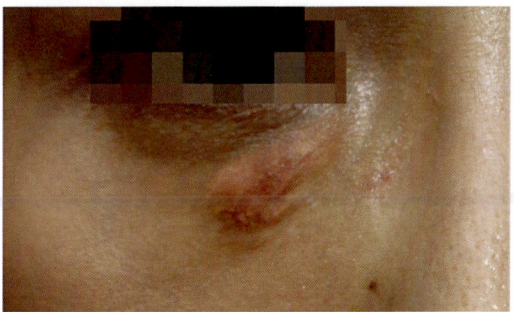

Fig. 1.8 The collagen filler. The collagen filler was injected to correct a tear trough. A hard particle is visible through the 3 months after the injection

Table 1.4   Etiology of infection

Cause	Injection kit contamination
	Septic condition
	Ischemic state due to excessive injection
	Previous skin infection
	Patient's own habits

phenomenon, the number of injections should be minimized or the needle changed during multiple injections.

• Contaminated during preparation is possible. An aseptic procedure cannot be overemphasized.

• Filler injections should be avoided in areas of previous skin infection or inflammation.
• Patients should be instructed not to compress, massage, or repeatedly touch the injection site.

The greatest proportion of infections occur after ischemic vascular compromise. Thus, treatment should be performed immediately when erythema persists for longer than 2 days and infection signs are present.

1.5.1   Symptoms

Infections are categorized as vascular compromise or general. Infections induced by ischemic changes are usually due to excessive filler injection. Erythema could be the natural course after injection because of circulation disturbances. If the skin can be stretched enough to withstand the pressure, the erythema disappears because of microcirculation improvements. However, if the skin cannot withstand the pressure, the erythema persists.

If erythema persists and an infection occurs after 48 hours, the cause of infection is a microcirculation problem; if an infection occurs without persistent erythema, it is likely to be a general infection. Both cases show signs of infection after 48 hours. Time variations occur according to compression severity. In cases of severe vascular compromise, infection sign might occur 36 hours. If it is not severe, infection signs might occur minimally after 72 hours. General infections tend to occur 2–5 days after injection because of the incubation period. However, if infection occurs before 72 hours, it is likely because of ischemic problem; if it occurs after 72 hours, it is likely due to a general infection (Figs. 1.9, 1.10, and 1.11).

Infection onset time is very important for distinguishing the cause of an infection. Causes of infection onset occurring before or after 72 hours are detailed as follows (Table 1.5).

1.5.2 Treatment

Minor infections would be cured by preventive antibiotics, but if the filler is contaminated, it

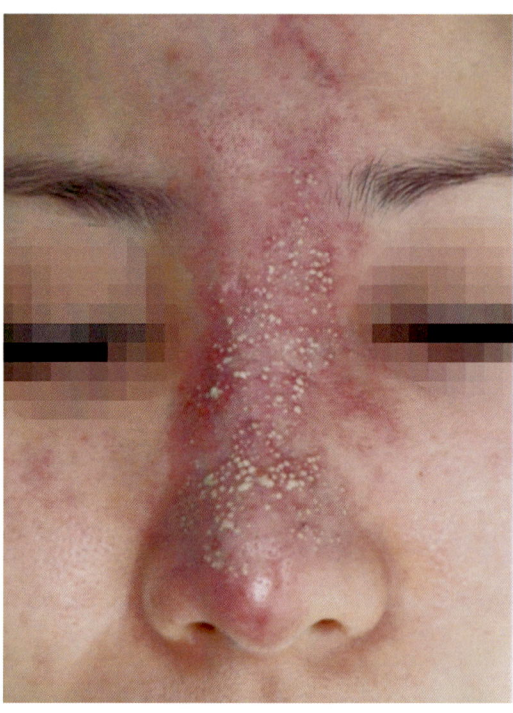

Fig. 1.10 Ischemic change and infection after hyaluronic acid filler injection. Infection after hyaluronic acid filler injection into the nose. An ischemic change and multiple pustules are visible

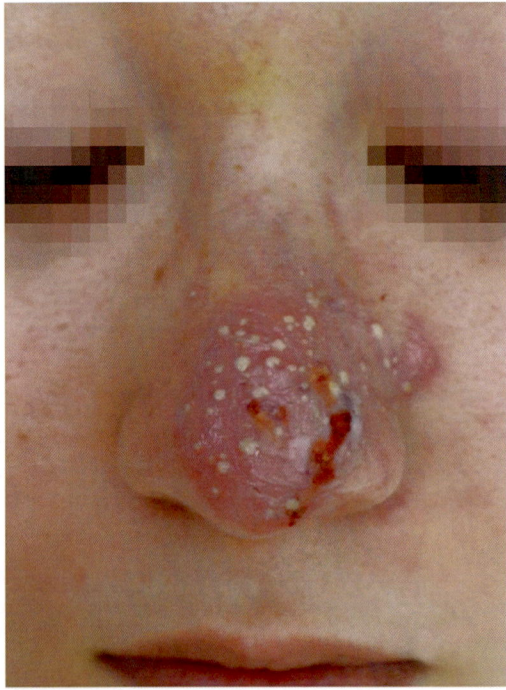

Fig. 1.9 Ischemic necrosis after hyaluronic acid filler injection. Four days after hyaluronic acid filler injection into the nasal tip, a classic ischemic necrosis pattern is visible; pustule appeared and spread after 48 hours

must be removed. Once the filler is determined to be contaminated, it should be treated as an infected foreign body. Antibiotics cannot reach the pathogen because the filler acts as a barrier and prolongs the infection. Thus, if there is any suspicion of infection, potent antibiotics like quinolone are needed; if there are signs of a prolonged infection, the filler must be removed. We recommend filler removal and immediate antibiotics administration if any signs of infection are seen.

The most important step is removing the cause of the infection when it occurs due to ischemic change. Thus, the most important treatment is decompression. One concern is that the iatrogenic spread of infection after hyaluronidase injection might destroy the inflammatory wall. Thus, when we inject hyaluronidase, inject exact layer of filler exist, and also dilute half dose of normal saline to minimized connection of infection. Another important thing is minimizing the number of injections and tissue damage.

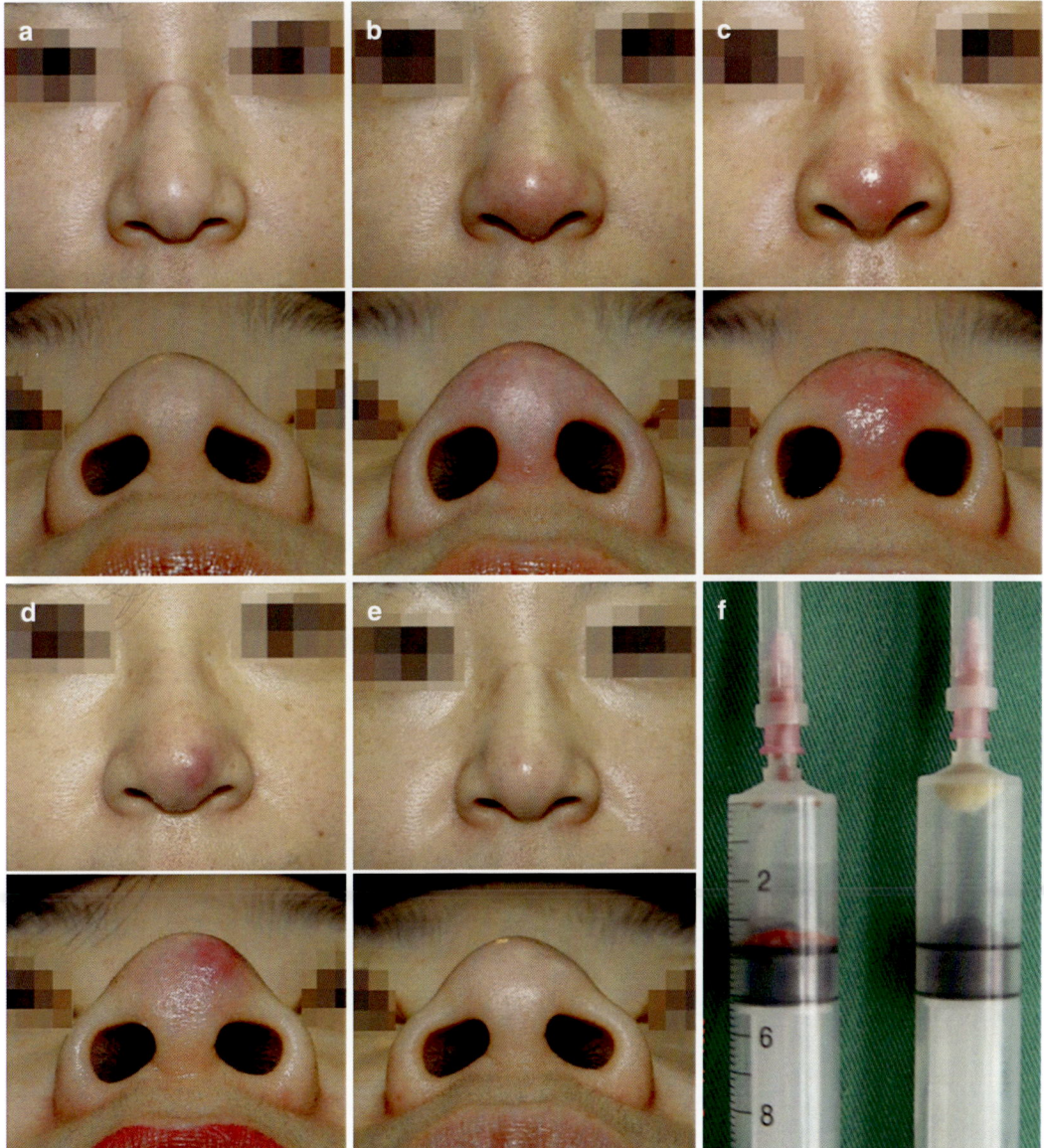

Fig. 1.11 Signs of general infection after polyacrylamide gel filler injection. Infection signs are seen 5 days after polyacrylamide gel filler injection. Despite treatment by systemic antibiotics, the localized infection remained. The filler and pus were aspirated by negative pressure aspiration. (**a**) View prior to polyacrylamide gel injection. (**b**) Immediately after injection. (**c**) Five days after injection with systemic antibiotics applied. (**d**) Three weeks after injection, signs of a localized infection were seen. The filler was removed by negative pressure aspiration. (**e**) Six months after filler removal. (**f**) Removed pus and filler

Antibiotics comprise the basic treatment of infection. A quinolone series are most commonly used, but a cephalosporin series is sufficient enough for mild infection. Intravenous administration is considered in severe cases, but oral administration is usually recommended. Antibiotics comprise supportive treatment to reduce pathogen spreading. In cases of ischemic status, the microcirculation is disturbed so antibiotic delivery to the infected lesion also tends to be low. Thus, directly removing the pustule and saving the damaged tissue are much more important than antibiotics.

Table 1.5 Cause of infection

Before 72 hours	Previous infection (dermatitis, acne) aggravated
	Disturbance of microcirculation by filler compression
	Immune disturbance
After 72 hours	Contaminated filler
	Prolonged inoculation time due to prophylactic antibiotic administration
	Infection occurred after injection (patient habit)

Pustules appear 48 hours after injection and spreading and become aggravated when infection occurs. Pustules appear because of breaching of the skin defense mechanism by ischemic damage and normal flora changes to toxic pathogens. Pustule treatment should include careful drainage. "Careful" means removing the pustule while damaging the adjacent tissue as little as possible. This adjacent tissue should not be destroyed because it would normalize after pustule removal. These tissues are fragile because of the microcirculation disturbance. Strong manipulation would lead to skin elimination, scars, and tissue loss. Thus, careful manipulation with gentle pressure is required to remove pus located at the subcutaneous layer.

After 48 hours, the pustule may be aggravated, so twice-daily dressing changes and pustule drainage are required to prevent tissue damage. We must drain the pustule first and apply antiseptic and Vaseline ointment gauze to prevent wound drying. Vaseline ointment prevents the gauze from sticking to the wound to prevent skin damage during removal. Applying an antiseptic such as povidone-iodine can be toxic to the wound, so consider its application in cases of severe infection.

It is very important that the wound not be dried. Wounds tend to dry out when a pustule is not removed properly or a wound dressing is not applied. When a wound dries, pus with discharge changes to a harder tissue scab. This scab tissue disturbs pus draining and wound healing. Thus, it is very important that the wound not to be dried, and once a scab appears, it should be removed very carefully using antiseptics such as hydrogen peroxide.

When applying gauze, it must not be compressed, as there are no benefits to a compressed wound.

If dressing and infection control are performed properly, then wounds likely heal within 7 days. After 7 days, hyperpigmentation tends to occur because of the tissue damage. Within 2 months, the hyperpigmentation might be aggravated, but after 3–4 months of ultraviolet (UV) protection, the pigmentation is likely to normalize. Thus, the application of UV protection cream and avoidance of laser treatment is recommended at the early stage.

Recently, a few novel treatments such as stem cell transplantation, platelet-rich protein (PRP), and epidermal growth factor (EGF) have been applied, but such treatments are not recommended during the infectious stage. These treatments might help wound healing.

1.6   Skin Necrosis

Skin necrosis is one of the tragic complications of filler injection. Detailed information about this will be described in Chap. 5.

1.6.1   Cause

Injected fillers disturb the circulation and skin necrosis results from ischemic damage. Ischemic damage causes infection and progression to infectious necrosis. The most mild phenomenon is erythema, while the most severe is skin necrosis.

1.6.2   Symptoms

Erythema is earliest symptom of skin necrosis. Blanching may be easily missed and easy to ignore because it tends to redden immediately. Local anesthetic creams or injections tend to make skin whiter than the surrounding areas. The important thing to note is that, after being reddish, instead of normalizing, the skin tends to develop a red wine color. This is the first symptom of disturbed circulation. This symptom fades gradually within 48 hours or rapidly progresses within 6 hours.

Reduced circulation causes ischemic damage and the tendency to progress to liquefaction and permanent damage. At this moment, the normal defense mechanisms might fail, and normal flora of the skin attacks then progresses to infectious necrosis. This usually starts within 48 hours, but severe compression could become evident within 36 hours.

Infectious necrosis begins with pus at the hair follicle; if it is unable to drain, the infection spreads to the subcutaneous tissue and aggravates the necrosis. A depressed scar may then form because of subcutaneous tissue destruction.

The red wine color indicates severe damage, while vasodilation appears red and orange. The wound is likely to be a scab because of dryness if a proper dressing cannot prevent wound drying. Pus under a scab tends to indicate more severe damage.

After infectious necrosis, permanent skin damage can occur. Scar tissues form at the skin damage site and affect the adjacent tissues by a process called scar contracture.

1.6.3 Treatment

Determining the stage of necrosis and responding quickly lead to a better prognosis. Decompression is the principle of necrosis treatment, and proper decompression determines the prognosis. When proper decompression is performed, then proper infection control is possible.

Severe necrosis does not occur when proper treatment is provided at the stage of ischemic necrosis or infectious necrosis. However, if necrosis occurred because of delayed treatment, there is a need to consider adjuvant therapy such as stem cell treatment, PRP, EGF, and polydeoxyribonucleic acid for wound healing.

Wide debridement or skin grafting could expedite wound healing, but it is not recommended because of the risk of disastrous aesthetic consequences.

1.7 Vascular Obstruction

Vascular obstruction results in localized or widespread phenomena. Severe complications such as blindness and cerebral embolism might happen due to extensive vascular obstructions.

1.7.1 Etiology

Localized vascular obstruction is usually caused by compression rather than filler embolism. In such cases, it is usually not affected by main vessels; rather, it is affected by small vessels and the vascular network, which is more superficial than the subcutaneous tissue and tends to be compressed.

When the main vessels are obstructed, symptoms tend to be more extensive and affected where the vessels are arborized. Main vessel obstructions are caused by emboli or compression. Main vessel obstructions also tend to be compressed, but they are usually located in the deeper subcutaneous layer, and vessel blood pressure is higher and less subjective to compressive obstruction.

The most serious problem is when fillers are injected directly to vessels and emboli run to the ocular vessels or brain vessels. If filler is injected with enough pressure to regurgitate, filler emboli run to ocular arteries or brain arteries. Table 1.6 demonstrates the risk factors of filler emboli.

The possibility of filler injection into a vessel is higher when the needle diameter is smaller. This is the same mechanism as with intravenous injection procedure, in which it is easier to inject into a vein with smaller needle. Thus, the injection of filler with a small-diameter needle could create an embolism because of the ease of injecting into a vessel and the relative higher pressure to extrude the filler.

Table 1.6 Risk factors of filler embolism

Higher-risk factors	Smaller needle diameter (smaller than 27G)
	High-pressure injection
	Compression where there is bleeding
	Injection into a highly vascular area

1.7.2 Symptoms

1.7.2.1 Localized Vascular Occlusion

Localized vascular occlusion usually occurs because of subcutaneous vascular network compression by the filler injection. Symptoms are localized, and the most severely compressed region tends to be the most reddish. The extent of redness depends on compression severity. Such areas tend to become blanched immediately. Localized vascular network compression results in blanching ischemic change, which promotes vasodilating mediators such as histamine release and color changes to red and a red wine color. If the pressure does not subside, infectious necrosis develops after 48 hours.

1.7.2.2 Extensive Vascular Occlusion

Extensive vascular occlusion occurs when the main vessels are obstructed by compression or embolism. It affects deeper vessels than in localized occlusion cases. It appears as the vessels are arborized. This is because relatively larger vessels are first affected, followed by other branched vessels. This is likely to feature inflammation at the injection site but might affect ischemic damage at distant lesions. It is likely to feature more extensive blanching lesions compared to localized occlusions and have a reticular pattern because of the vascular territory. If it continues, compression is likely to progress to the infectious stage.

1.7.2.3 Distant Vessel Obstruction

Vessel obstruction at a distant location occurs when filler is injected into anatomically well-known arteries. The locations of the injection site and affected arteries are described in Table 1.7.

Table 1.7 Arteries associated with filler embolism

Nasolabial fold correction	Lateral nasal artery, facial artery
Nose augmentation	Dorsal nasal artery
Temple augmentation	Superficial temporal artery
Glabella, forehead	Supratrochlear artery, supraorbital artery
Cheek	Transverse facial artery

Filler injected into these arteries could overcome arterial pressure and regurgitate to the ophthalmic arteries or cerebral arteries and cause blindness or brain infarction. Complication symptoms can be seen immediately such as blindness or neurological signs and should be treated immediately because these are the most emergent situations. However, in reality, there are no specific treatments for these situations. We will discuss this in detail in Chap. 6.

1.7.3 Treatment

1.7.3.1 Localized Vessel Obstruction Treatment

Prognosis depends on how fast decompensation can occur. When injecting hyaluronic acid filler, hyaluronidase should be injected to provide decompensation. Hyaluronidase contains 1500 IU in each vial and is usually mixed with 1–1.5 cc of normal saline. When ischemic complications occur, the injection of one vial of hyaluronidase is recommended. For example, when compression of the nasal tip is suspected after the injection of 0.1–0.2 cc of filler, 0.5 cc of hyaluronidase should be administered and massaged very gently. Massage is needed to spread the hyaluronidase because the filler will not degrade otherwise. However, it should be done very gently to prevent the destruction of destroy fragile tissues.

A problem occurs in cases of delayed detection of ischemic changes and the progression to necrosis. Nevertheless, we must inject hyaluronidase. However, we should carefully inject hyaluronidase in cases of wound infection because the infection might spread. Thus, it is recommended that a half dose of normal saline be mixed with hyaluronidase and be injected at the exact filler location. The pustule should be removed before the hyaluronidase injection and care taken to prevent damage to the normal fragile tissue.

Even damaged tissues should be preserved whenever possible rather than debrided or removed. These fragile tissues act as a framework of the wound healing process, and the viability of this tissue is important for prognosis. Thus, it is important to preserve viable tissue whenever possible, remove the pustules very carefully, and cover the wound with Vaseline gauze. As mentioned before, if the wound is dried, a scab is created, and pus cannot drain, so a depressed scar would occur; thus, a wound should not be allowed to dry.

Antiseptics such as povidone-iodine are quite toxic and should be used minimally in cases of definite infectious signs.

When applying a dressing, clean all exudates and drain the pustules, and then cover the wound with Vaseline gauze to prevent the dried gauze and exudate from sticking together. Changing of the Vaseline gauze should be done until there are no pustule and exudate. If the infection has subsided, the dressing should be minimal to promote wound healing. Dressings should cover the wound widely to protect the fragile tissues.

Dressing should be done until complete re-epithelization occurs. Patients should be educated about how to prevent hyperpigmentation. Post-inflammatory hyperpigmentation might occur until 2 months, but it usually recovers to normal. However, UV exposure can prolong hyperpigmentation, so it is important to apply UV protection cream.

1.7.3.2 Extensive Vascular Obstruction Treatment

When suspected, immediate decompression and aseptic dressing can be used to achieve a full recovery. Aggressive treatment might lead to better results than localized compression because it uses collateral circulation.

1.7.3.3 Distant Vascular Obstruction Treatment

Visual disturbance or cerebral infarction patients should be transferred immediately. Retrobulbar hyaluronidase injections were recently proposed for treatment, but they are not yet definite. Ocular massage has also been proposed, but scientific evidence of this is lacking. We will discuss multiple treatments in Chap. 6.

1.8 Migration

Filler usually remains where it is injected, but it can migrate. This phenomenon can be divided into immediate migration and delayed migration.

1.8.1 Cause

1.8.1.1 Immediate Migration

Immediate migration is usually a result of medical malpractice, i.e., a high-pressure injection without external guide. That means that we can prevent filler migration by making a guide with external pressing.

When filler is injected, it is likely to move to the tissue with the lowest resistance. This happens when the injection is highly pressurized. For example, when filler is injected to correct nasolabial folds, it tends to spread above the nasolabial fold because those tissues are softer. If the injected pressure is higher, filler might enter the posterior part of the maxillary bone. Thus, nasolabial fold correction should be performed while pressing on the areas to which spreading is not desired. The clinician must check every minute whether the filler is properly lifting the soft tissues.

Amazingly, filler is sometimes found in distant places. One patient who underwent nasolabial fold correction displayed swelling of the upper lips after injection. Apparently a tunnel was created through the subcutaneous layer through which the injected filler migrated. The filler was immediately removed from the upper lip, but the rest of the filler had to be removed as well since it was likely to migrate through the tunnel over time.

Thus, it is very important to check between the procedures and provide guidance with external handling. Injections made with smaller needles require more pressure, so they should be performed more carefully.

Tissue density is also important. Soft tissues tend to have high lifting capacity with low injection pressure, which minimizes the possibility of migration. However, very dense tissues require high pressure and a larger volume to create lift, which increases the risk of migration.

1.8.1.2 Delayed Migration

Patient Manipulation

The most common reason of filler migration is patient manipulation. Filler is basically viscous material that can change shape when compressed. Patient may attempt to mold the area as the doctor does immediately after the injection, which may induce migration.

A depressive finding follows filler migration because of loss of the initial lifted volume. This might occur with highly cohesive fillers because filler should be well integrated with the tissue rather than cohesive with itself (Fig. 1.12).

The nose, nasolabial fold, forehead, and chin are the places that patients are likely to compress. Thus, after filler injection, it is quite important to warn patients that it might migrate when compressed (Figs. 1.13, 1.14, and 1.15).

Migration due to Filler Properties

Migration due to properties of different fillers usually occurs at the nose or chin, where it is expected to maintain shape against high pressure. When soft fillers are used in these areas, the initial shape is good, but the look spreads and widens over time. Injected filler in the chin area tends to migrate with mentalis muscle action (Fig. 1.16).

This phenomenon can also be seen at the nose with the use of soft fillers. The nose is usually divided into the nasal root, supratip depression, and nasal tip (Fig. 1.17).

Over time, filler injected into the supratip depression tended to migrate to the nasal

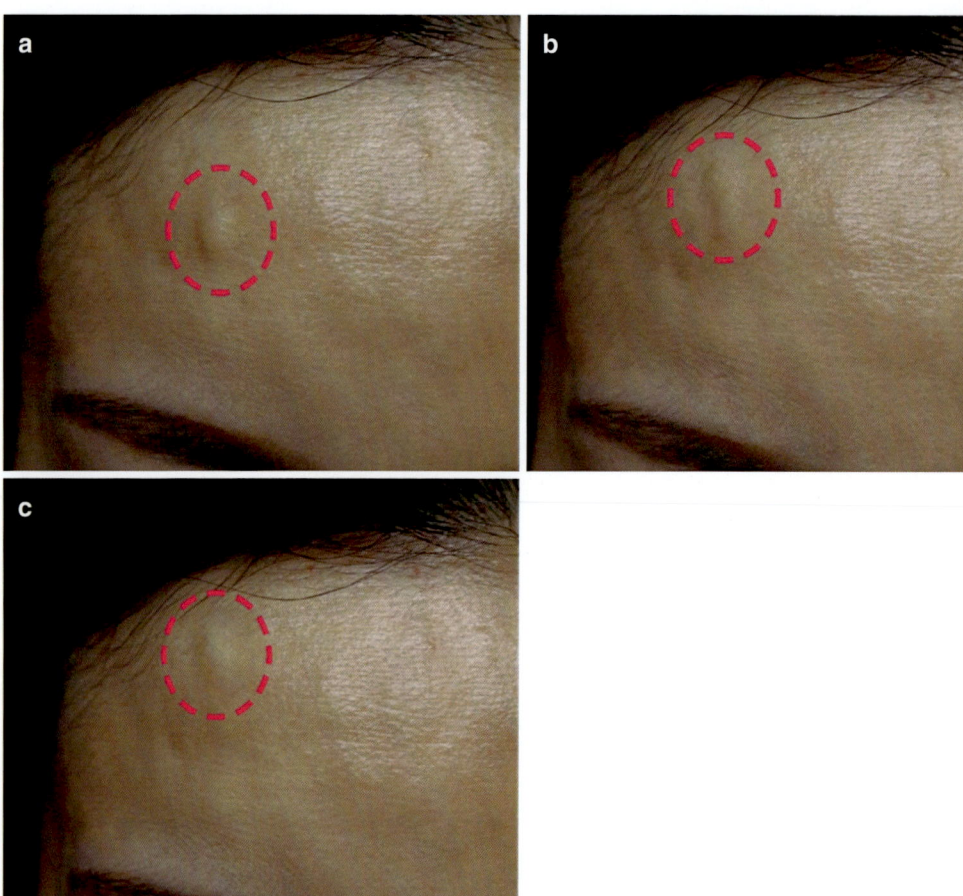

Fig. 1.12 Migration of hyaluronic acid filler – the tunneling phenomenon. Seven months after forehead augmentation by hyaluronic acid filler injection, a highly cohesive filler tends to migrate through the tunnel. (**a**) Filler seen at the lowest part of the subcutaneous layer tunnel. (**b**) Fillers seen at the diffuse part of the tunnel. (**c**) Filler seen at the highest part of the tunnel. Filler can migrate easily by patient manipulation

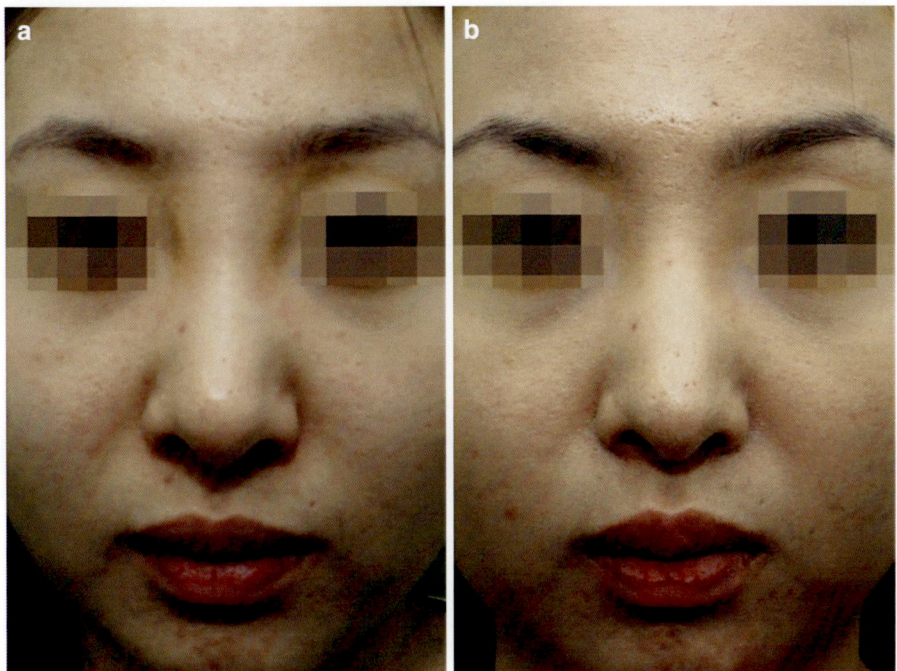

Fig. 1.13 Migration and removal of hyaluronic acid filler. The hyaluronic acid filler migrated to the nasal root and looked wide, so it was removed. (**a**) Before removal. (**b**) After removal

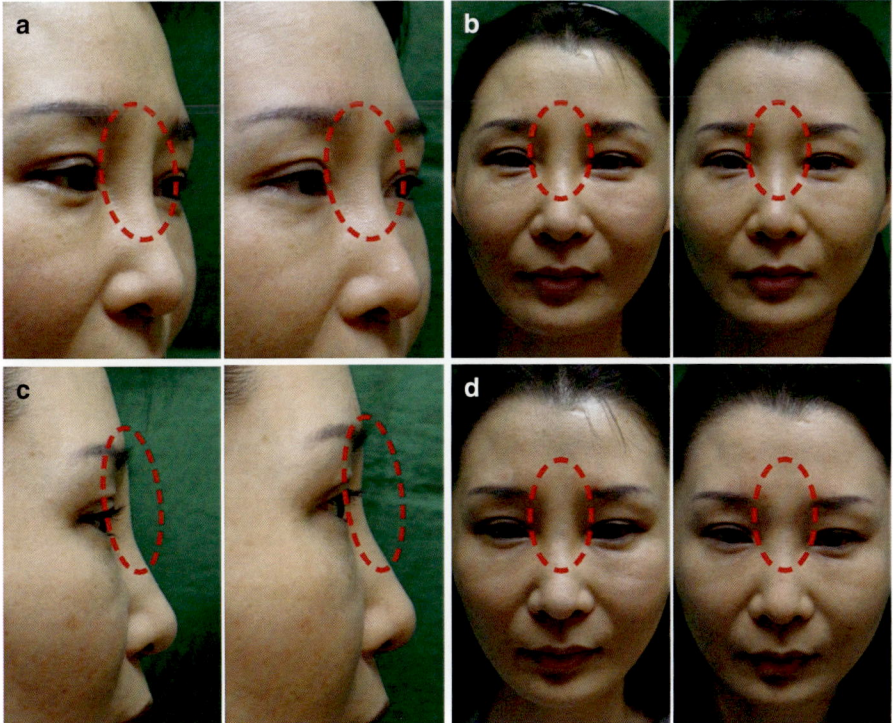

Fig. 1.14 Migration and removal of polyacrylamide gel filler. Images of polyacrylamide gel filler having migrated to the nasal root and 1 month after its removal. (**a**) Before and after removal. (**b**) Before and after removal. (**c**) Before and after removal. (**d**) Before and after removal

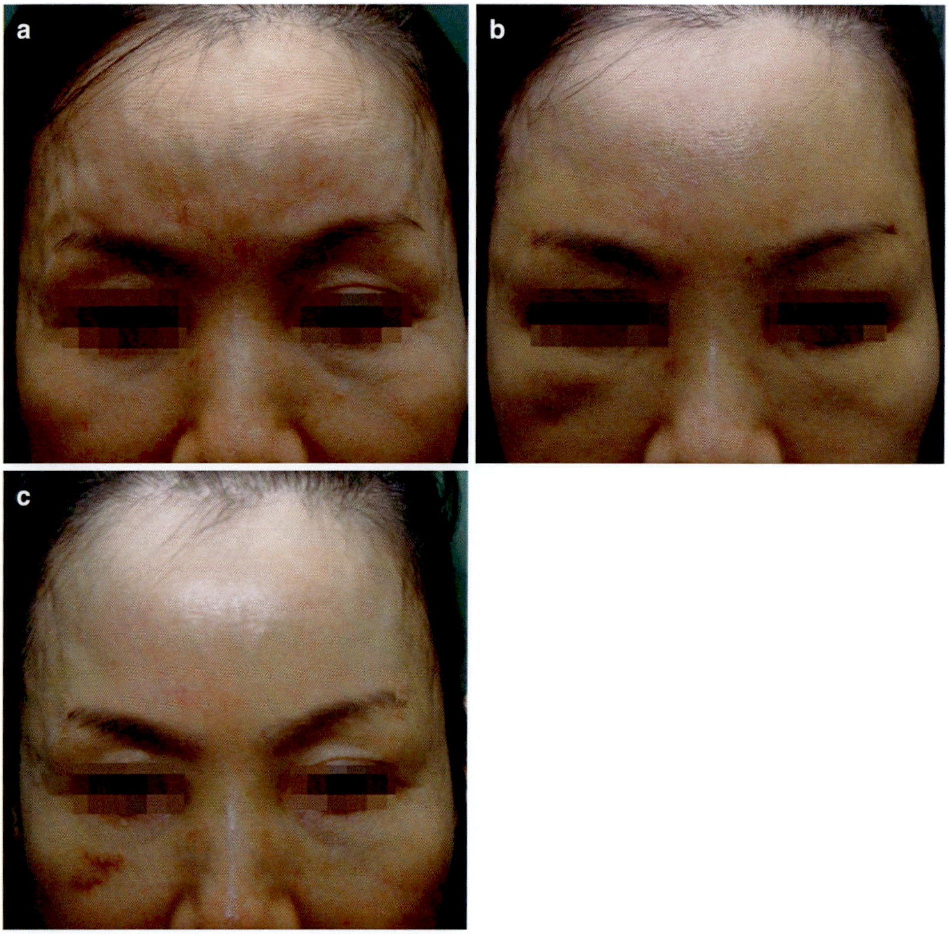

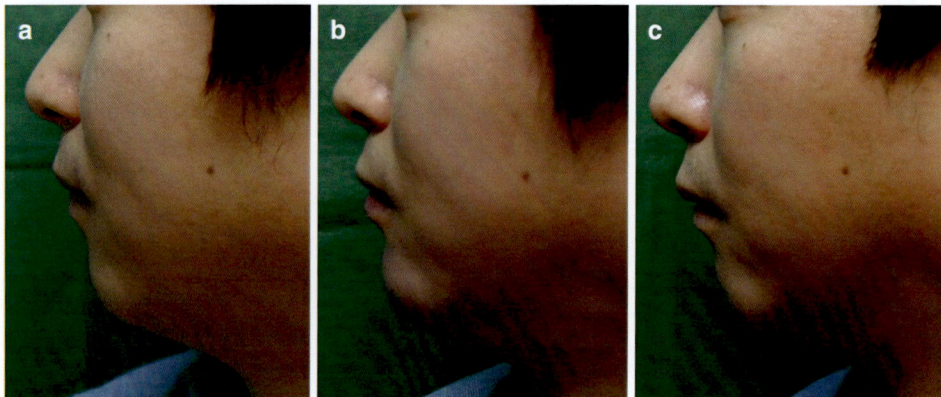

Fig. 1.15 Migration and removal of polyacrylamide gel filler – the tunneling phenomenon. Polyacrylamide gel filler migrated upward after patient self-massage. When the migrating occurred, a crowned appearance developed. The filler was removed using negative pressure needle aspiration and squeezing. (**a**) Filler migration appearance. (**b**) Four days after filler removal by negative pressure aspiration. (**c**) Two weeks after removal

Fig. 1.16 Migration of hyaluronic acid filler. The anterior chin was augmented by hyaluronic acid filler, and the immediate postinjection view demonstrated good augmentation. After 2 months, the filler disappeared and migrated because of its properties and the mentalis muscle action. (**a**) Before injection. (**b**) Immediately after injection. (**c**) Two months after injection

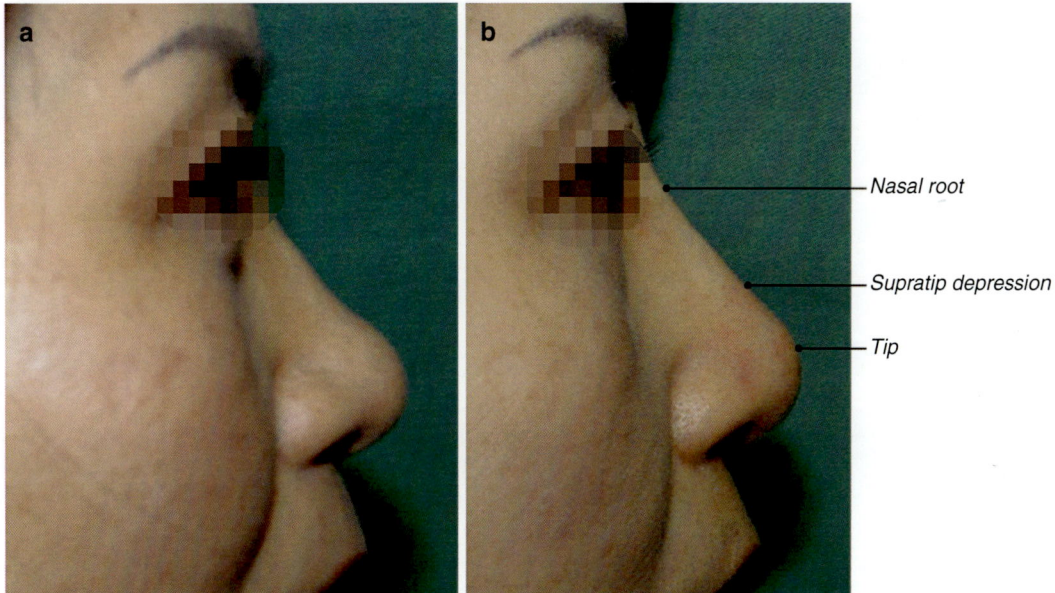

Fig. 1.17 Filler injection site on the nose. (**a**) Preinjection. (**b**) Postinjection: nasal root, supratip depression, nasal tip

root or nasal tip. This phenomenon occurred because this area was thinner than the soft tissue at the nasal root or tip. This phenomenon occurs gradually and can be seen by permanent fillers compared to hyaluronic acid fillers (Fig. 1.18).

Horizontal and perpendicular migration can occur. This is usually seen at the nasal tip, i.e., the first injected area, which was superficial to the alar cartilage but migrated to the soft tissue. This might be seen when the skin is relatively not dense or a patient squeezes the nasal tip (Fig. 1.19).

Migration due to Muscle Action

Migration due to muscle action is typically seen when filler is injected into the forehead and frontalis muscle action and corrugator supercilii muscle action induces migration (Fig. 1.20).

Photograph should be taken of the patients making facial expressions. Irregularities in this area should be compared to this photograph, and botulinum toxin should be injected to correct the issue (Fig. 1.21).

1.9 Transparent Effect and Tyndall Effect

The transparent effect is that injected filler can be seen through thin skin. If the filler has color itself, it is likely to be visible. Colored fillers include calcium hydroxyapatite filler (white), collagen filler (yellow), and polycaprolactone filler (white) (Figs. 1.22, 1.23, 1.24, and 1.25).

Most fillers are colorless. In addition to a transparent effect, a Tyndall effect is visible.

★ Tyndall effect: Light scattering by particles in a colloid or very fine suspension. Fillers under the skin tend to scatter light and appear blue.

1.9.1 Cause

The Tyndall effect is seen when inject transparent filler is injected into the superficial layer of thin skin. The more filler is injected, the higher the risk of the Tyndall effect due to greater reflection of the medium. The only prevention consists of not injecting filler superficially and injecting only

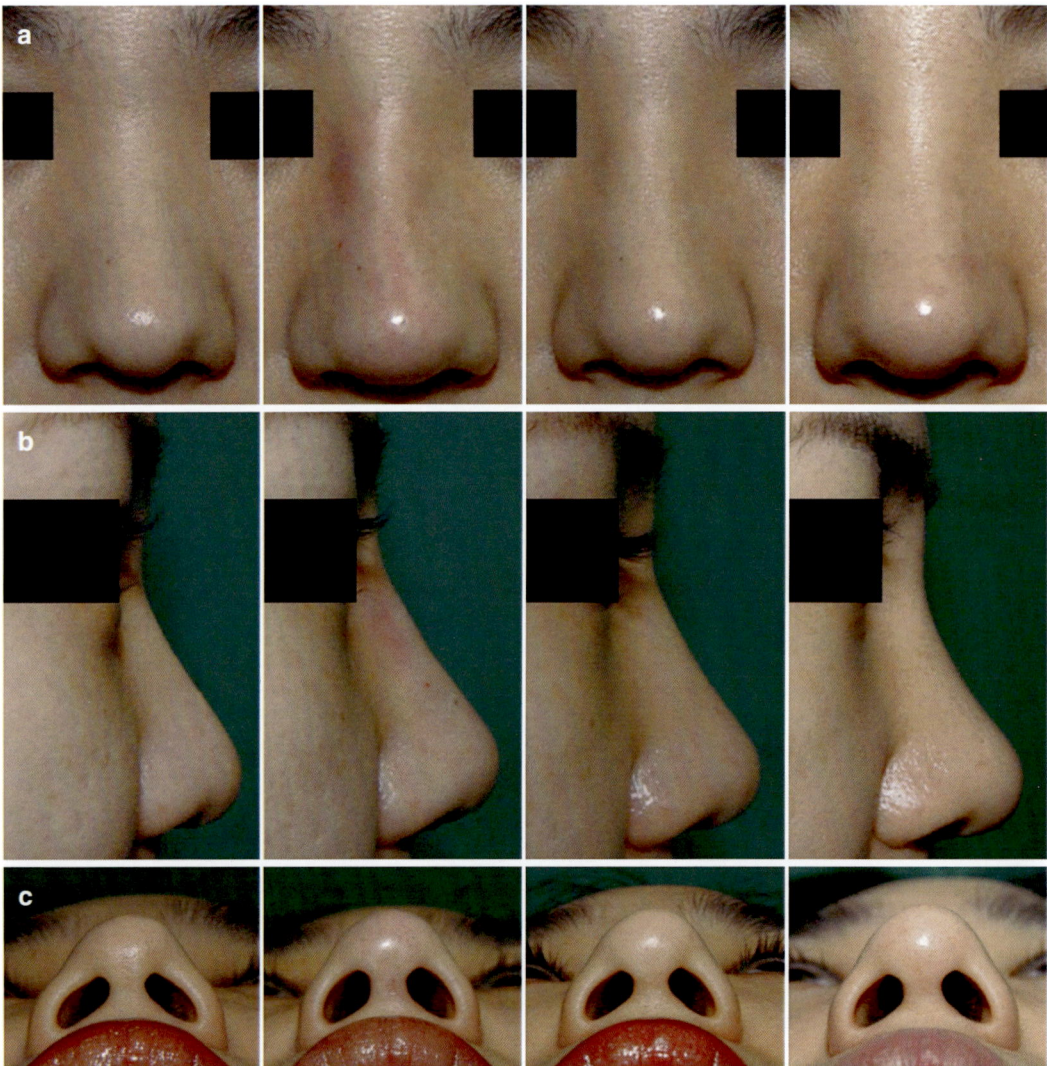

Fig. 1.18 Horizontal migration of polyacrylamide gel filler. Nasal shape changes occur over time after poly-acrylamide gel filler injection. Preinjection, immediate postinjection, 2 weeks postinjection, and 10 months postinjection views. The nose looks straight immediately 2 weeks after, but the filler migrated to the root resulting in a higher root area and migrated to the tip, resulting in a wider tip. (**a**) Frontal view: preinjection, immediately postinjection, 2 weeks postinjection, and 10 months postinjection. (**b**) Lateral view: preinjection, immediately postinjection, 2 weeks postinjection, and 10 months postinjection. (**c**) Worm's eye view: preinjection, immediately postinjection, 2 weeks postinjection, and 10 weeks postinjection

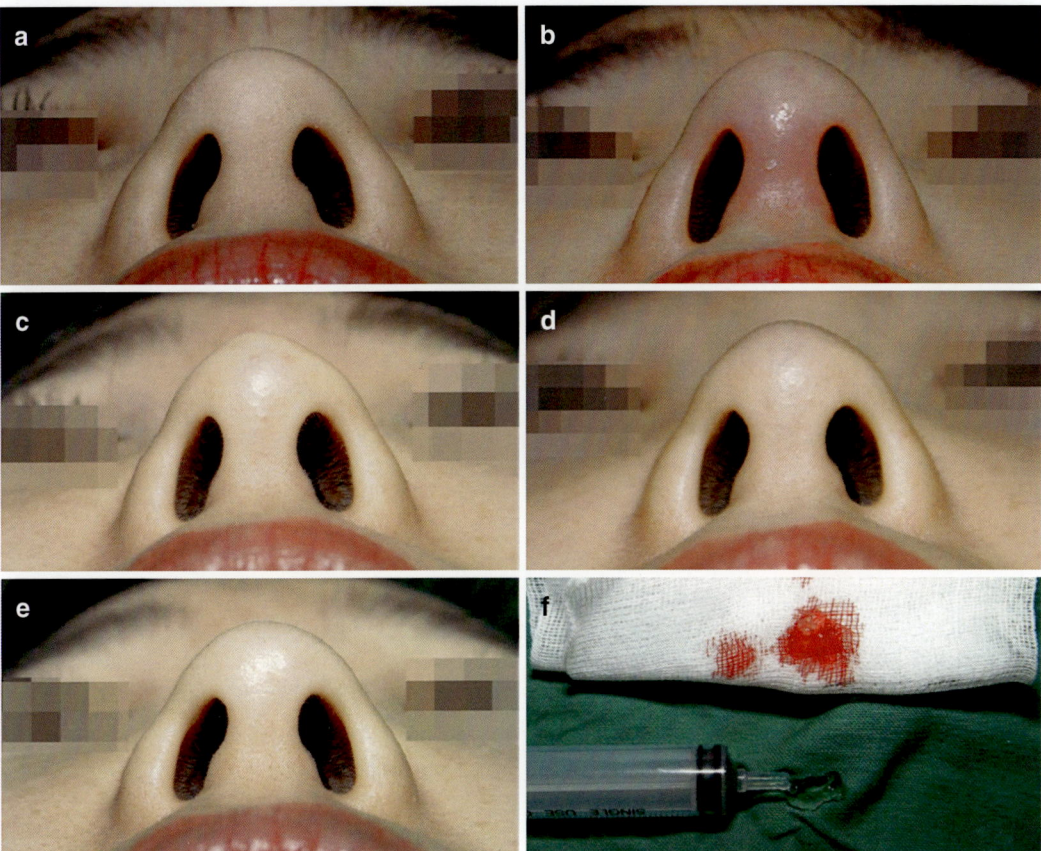

Fig. 1.19 Perpendicular migration and removal of poly-acrylamide gel filler. Nasal tip injection with polyacryl-amide gel filler, which was first injected onto the alar cartilage but migrated and was removed. (**a**) Preinjection. (**b**) Two weeks after injection. (**c**) Eight months after injection, when subcutaneous migration is visible. (**d**) Twenty-six months after injection, at which time more filler had migrated and the skin color had changed to a bluish color because of Tyndall effects. (**e**) Seventeen months after filler removal using negative pressure aspiration. (**f**) Polyacrylamide gel filler removed using negative pressure aspiration

small amounts of filler. Thus, clinicians must be careful about skin thickness and regulate the amount of filler used.

1.9.2   Location

The Tyndall effect can occur when filler is injected into thin skin, particularly in the pret-arsal area, tear trough, lips, and nose. The nose contains relatively thick skin, but when large volumes of filler are used, greater reflection of medium can occur.

The pretarsal region is where the Tyndall effect frequently occurs. For prevention, it is better to inject fillers into deeper layers than the orbicularis oculi muscle. Since the pretar-sal portion of the orbicularis oculi muscle is

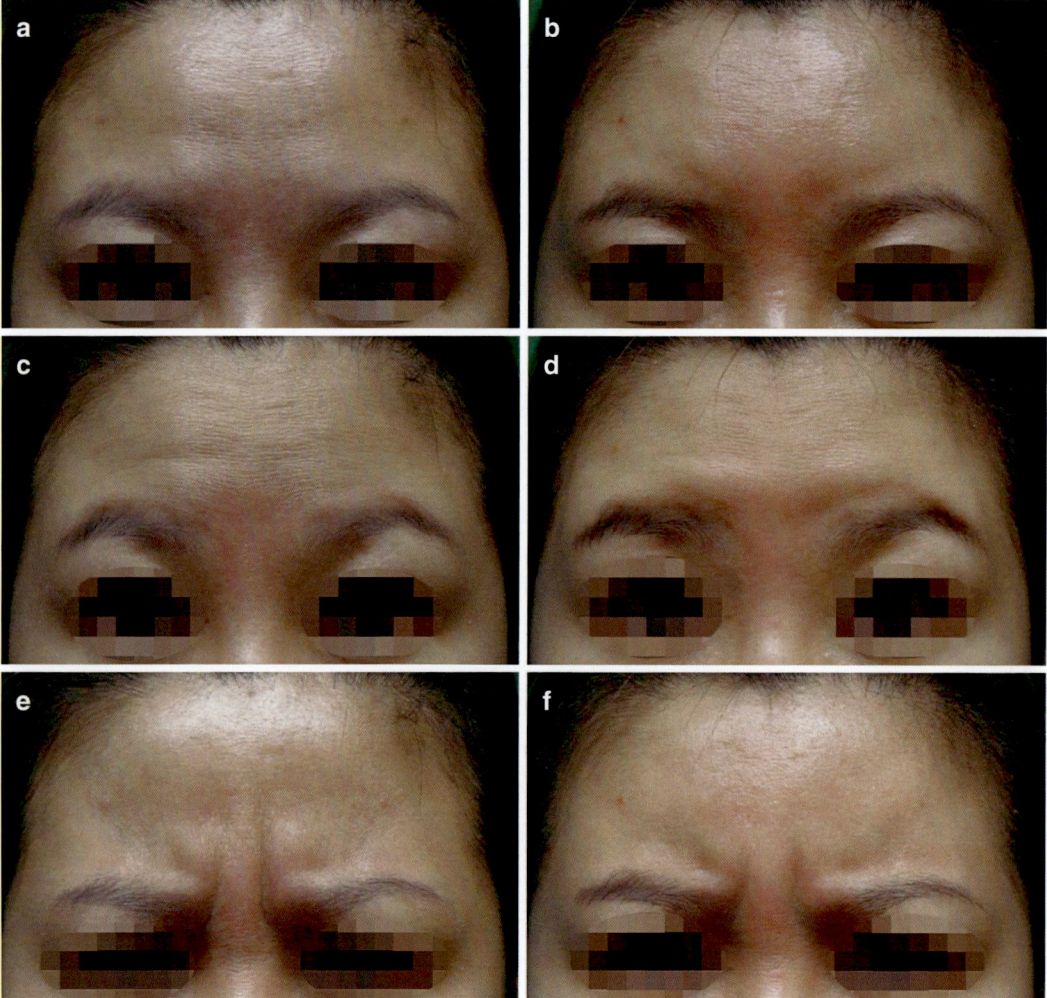

Fig. 1.20 Filler migration due to frontalis muscle and corrugator supercilii muscle action. Hyaluronic acid filler was injected into the forehead and migrated due to frontalis muscle action. (**a**, **b**) Preinjection and 1 month postinjection showing upward filler migration when the patient shows no expression. (**c**, **d**) Preinjection and 1 month postinjection showing migration with frontalis muscle action. (**e**, **f**) Preinjection and 1 month postinjection showing migration with corrugator supercilii muscle action

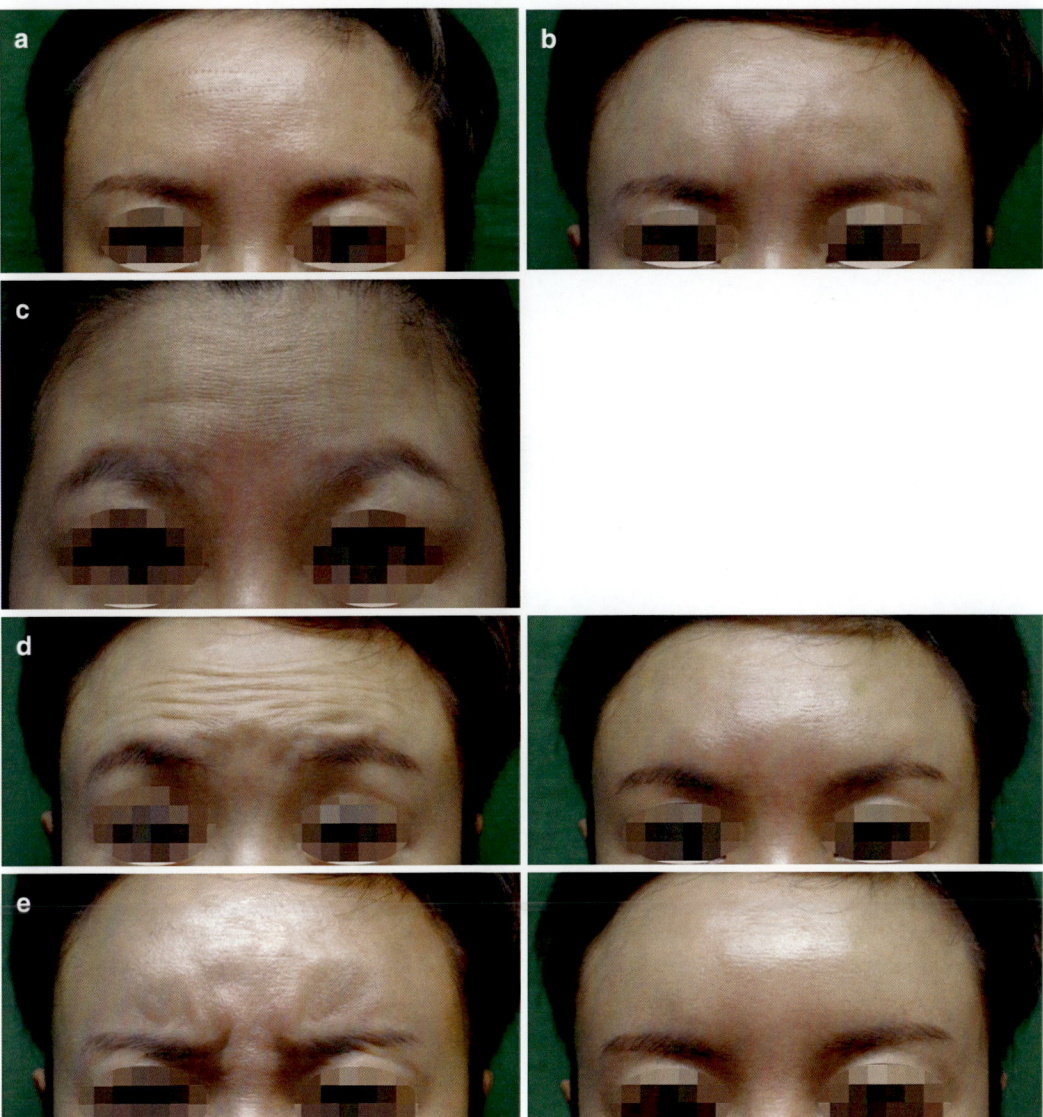

Fig. 1.21 Filler migration due to frontalis muscle and corrugator supercilii muscle actions. Two weeks after the hyaluronic acid filler was injected into the forehead, the irregularity was corrected. Botulinum toxin might be considered at the forehead filler injection area. (**a**) Preinjection. (**b**) Two weeks after forehead filler injection, the filler was seen to have migrated due to frontalis muscle and corrugator supercilii muscle actions. (**c**) One week after botulinum toxin was injected into the frontalis muscle and corrugator supercilii muscle to correct the irregularity. (**d**) Before botulinum toxin injection and 1 week after the frontalis muscle injection showing that the forehead wrinkling had improved. (**e**) Before botulinum toxin injection and 1 week after the corrugator supercilii muscle injection showing that the glabellar wrinkle had improved and the migration had disappeared

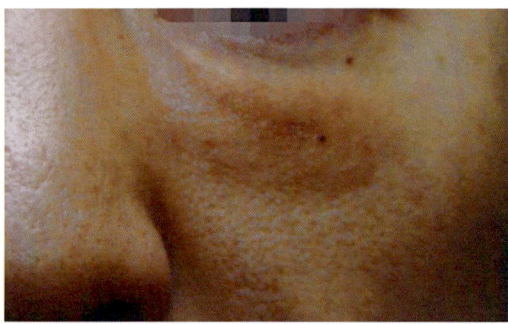

Fig. 1.22 Calcium hydroxyapatite filler transparent effect. White filler is visible through the thin skin after the injection of calcium hydroxyapatite filler to correct a tear trough deformity

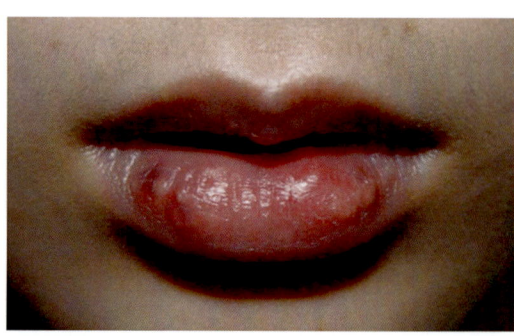

Fig. 1.25 The collagen filler transparent effect. The collagen filler injected into the lower lip appears as yellow areas

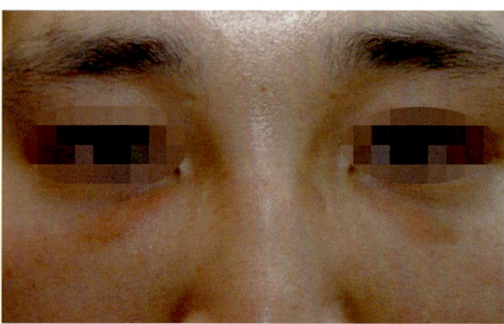

Fig. 1.23 Calcium hydroxyapatite filler transparent effect. Calcium hydroxyapatite filler injected to correct a tear trough deformity

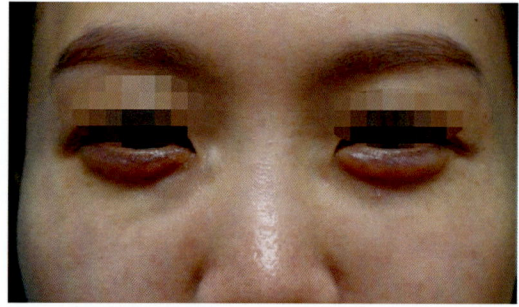

Fig. 1.26 Tyndall effect of the hyaluronic acid filler. Two weeks after pretarsal augmentation by the hyaluronic acid filler. A bluish Tyndall effect is visible

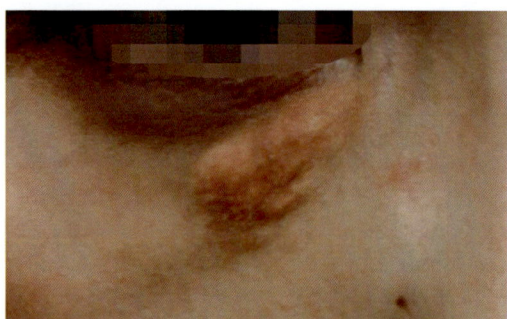

Fig. 1.24 The collagen filler transparent effect. Yellow filler can be seen through thin skin after the injection of the collagen filler to correct a tear trough deformity

very thin, one should inject the filler onto the tarsal plate. However, the filler could migrate to the subcutaneous layer, so it is important to warn patients about the Tyndall effect (Fig. 1.26).

To avoid the Tyndall effect at the tear trough, do not inject filler into the superficial layer; rather, inject it to correct the deep groove. Educate the patient about the Tyndall effect prior to making the injection (Fig. 1.27).

The Tyndall effect can occur at the nose after a superficial injection. Upon the injection of large volumes of filler, the Tyndall effect can occur. The dorsum of the nose is particularly susceptible because the skin there is relatively thinner and a large volume is injected. When injecting a large volume at the superficial nasal tip, the Tyndall effect might be seen. However, filler might migrate superficially when it is injected into the deep layer above the interdomal alar cartilage (Fig. 1.28).

The Tyndall effect might also occur at the lips because of thin skin and mucosa. When filler is injected into the submucous layer,

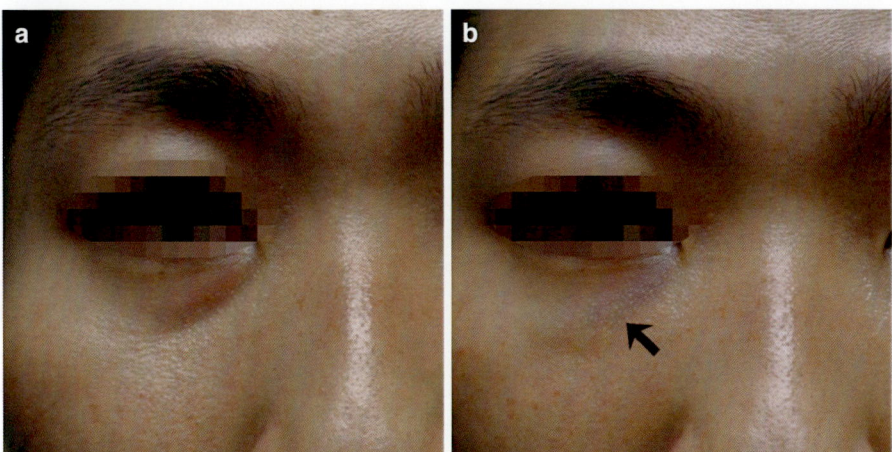

Fig. 1.27 Tyndall effect of hyaluronic acid filler. Two months after tear trough injection of hyaluronic acid filler, the tear trough was corrected, but the Tyndall effect occurred on the right side. (**a**) Preinjection. (**b**) Two months after the injection

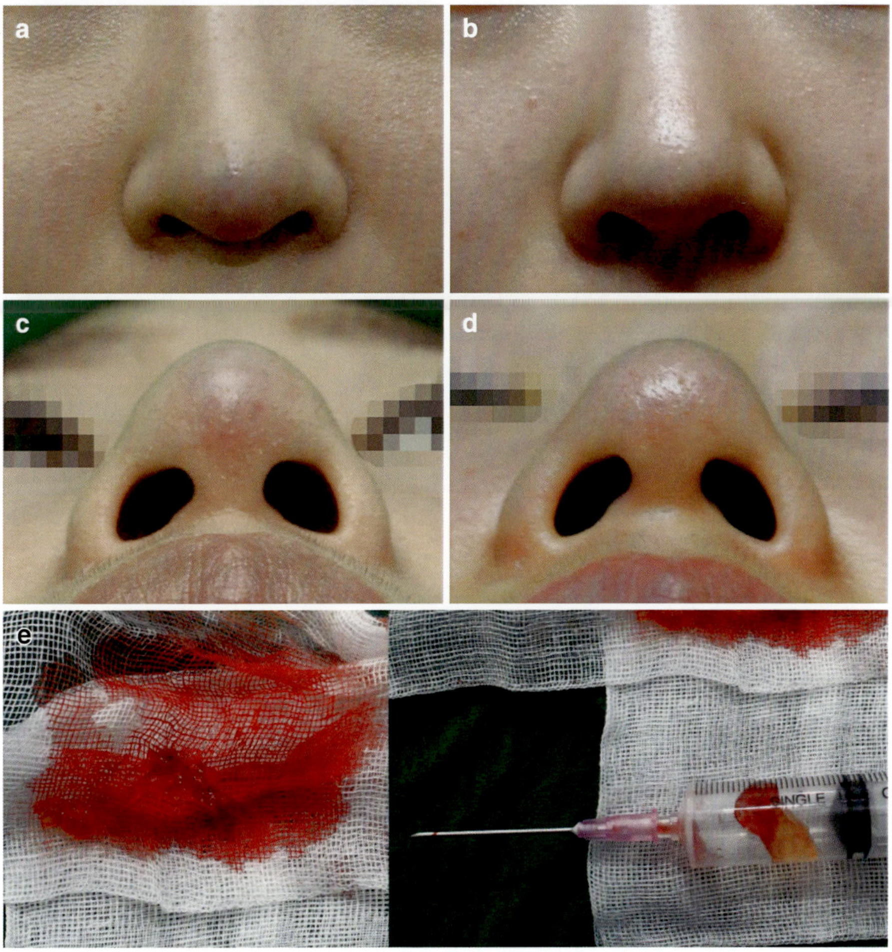

Fig. 1.28 Tyndall effect of polyacrylamide gel filler. Five years after polyacrylamide gel filler injection, the Tyndall effect is visible due to superficial migration. (**a**) Five years after polyacrylamide gel filler injection, a bluish color is seen. (**b**) After filler removal. (**c**) Worm's eye view of filler migration. (**d**) After removal. (**e**) Removed filler

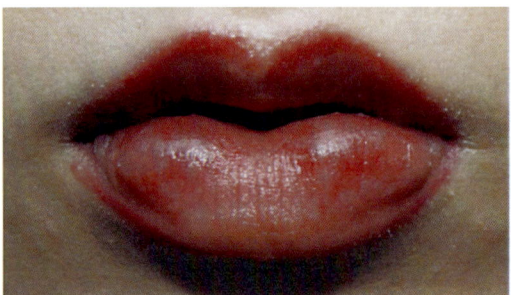

Fig. 1.29 Tyndall effect of hyaluronic acid filler. Two weeks after lip augmentation, the Tyndall effect is seen in the lower lip

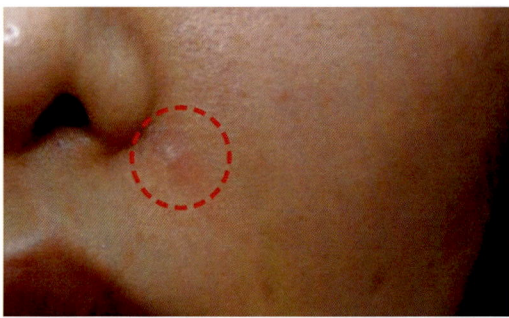

Fig. 1.30 Skin marking. Permanent skin marking occurring after superficial injection into the nasolabial fold

transparency is higher at the mucosa, making the Tyndall effect more common (Fig. 1.29).

1.9.3 Prevention and Treatment

Filler removal is key to treatment. Hyaluronic acid filler is removed by hyaluronidase, while colored fillers such as calcium hydroxyapatite filler, polycaprolactone filler, and the collagen filler and permanent fillers such as polyacrylamide gel filler should be removed by aspiration.

The Tyndall effect that occurs due to a large injection amount can be solved by reducing the amount.

To prevent the Tyndall effect and transparent effect, filler should be injected in small amounts and injected deeply in high-risk areas. Colored fillers should not be used in these areas. Patients should be warned when such fillers are used in high-risk areas.

1.10 Skin Marking

Skin marking is an extruded scar created by the filler injection due to extensive extension of the skin such as striae gravidarum. Less extension and excessive soothing like striae distensae appear when too much filler presses against superficial skin. If the pressure continues, a permanent scar may form (Fig. 1.30). If the filler contains hyaluronic acid, hyaluronidase can be used for degradation.

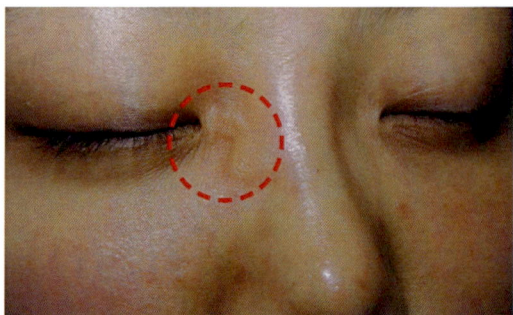

Fig. 1.31 Allergic reaction by polyacrylamide gel filler

1.11 Allergic Reactions

Allergic reaction can be seen immediate after filler injection (Fig. 1.31). Allergic reaction can be cured by steroid creams and/or steroid and antihistamine drugs (Fig. 1.32)

1.12 Filler-Induced Hypersensitivity Inflammation and Granuloma

Granuloma is the permanent tissue change that occurs after repetitive tissue reactions in which it becomes hard and solid. There are many assumptive causes, including filler toxicity (especially cross-linking agents), osmolarity, pH imbalance, and hyaluronic acid impurities. These complications are visible in the cheek, chin, nose, and periocular areas.

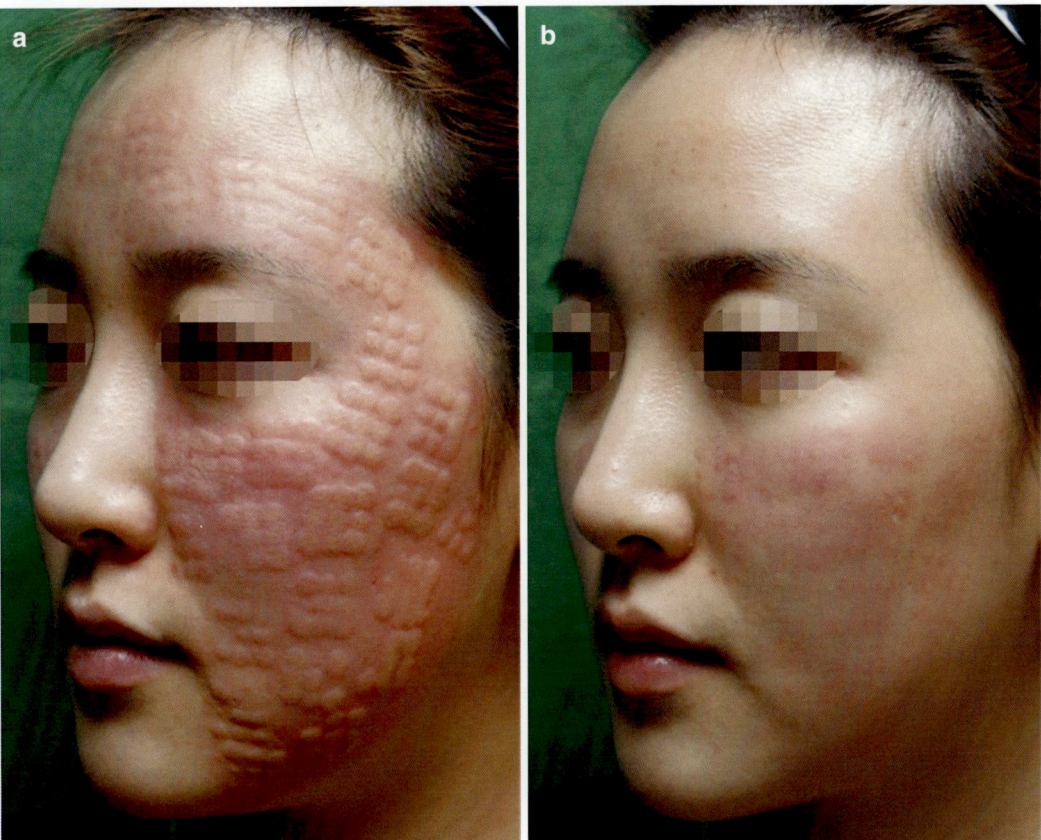

Fig. 1.32 Allergic reaction by hyaluronic acid filler. (**a**) Intradermal injection-induced allergic reaction, (**b**) One day after steroid cream applied

Clinical symptoms include repetitive swelling, flushing, pain at the injection site, and spreading to the surrounding areas. This is likely to subside with anti-inflammatory drug use, but since the tissue reactions continue, a hard solid nodule is likely to form that shows tenderness, compressive pain, or facial asymmetry.

A hypersensitivity reaction occurs when the patient is in an immunosuppressive state, tired, menstruating, or in an upper respiratory infection state. Thus, when a patient complains about repetitive swelling during such conditions, a filler-induced hypersensitivity reaction is likely the cause.

Cases have recently increased because of high doses of cross-linking agent or/and low-quality hyaluronic acid powder. We can assume that the manufacturing process would be a high potential cause of granuloma.

Granuloma is also likely to appear when a patient keeps touching the injected area because the injected filler is likely exposed to the adjacent tissue. This filler-induced hypersensitivity inflammation and granuloma will be described in Chap. 3.

Further Reading

1. Alijotas-Reig J, Fernandez-Figueras MT, Puig L. Late-onset inflammatory adverse reactions related to soft tissue filler injections. Clin Rev Allergy Immunol. 2013;45(1):97–108.
2. Alijotas-Reig J, Fernandez-Figueras MT, Puig L. Inflammatory, immune-mediated adverse reactions related to soft tissue dermal fillers. Semin Arthritis Rheum. 2013;43(2):241–58.
3. Constantine RS, Constantine FC, Rohrich RJ. The ever-changing role of biofilms in plastic surgery. Plast Reconstr Surg. 2014;133(6):865e–72e.

4. Fernandez-Cossio S, Castano-Oreja MT. Biocompatibility of two novel dermal fillers: histological evaluation of implants of a hyaluronic acid filler and a polyacrylamide filler. Plast Reconstr Surg. 2006;117(6):1789–96.

5. Funt D, Pavicic T. Dermal fillers in aesthetics: an overview of adverse events and treatment approaches. Plast Surg Nurs. 2015;35(1):13–32.

6. Lemperle G, Gauthier-Hazan N, Wolters M, Eisemann-Klein M, Zimmermann U, Duffy DM. Foreign body granulomas after all injectable dermal fillers: part 1. Possible causes. Plast Reconstr Surg. 2009;123(6):1842–63.

7. Ono S, Ogawa R, Hyakusoku H. Complications after polyacrylamide hydrogel injection for soft-tissue augmentation. Plast Reconstr Surg. 2010;126(4):1349–57.

Hyaluronic Acid Filler and Hyaluronidase

Hyaluronic acid (HA) filler is a soft-tissue filler that is used in >80% of the market. Since the US Food and Drug Administration approved Restylane® (Q Med Company, Sweden) in 2003, HA fillers made of cross-linked HA have been commonly used because of their superior safety compared to other PMMA, PAAG, PCL, and PLLA fillers. Another advantage of HA fillers is that they can be dissolved in case of unexpected results, such as undesired outcomes or complications.

Clinicians should be educated about the fundamental manufacturing process and basic properties of hyaluronic acid fillers to prepare them for cases of complications. In this chapter, we will discuss the basic properties and associated complications of HA fillers and describe hyaluronidase, the most important drug used to treat such complications.

and synthesized daily. Hyaluronic acid molecule structures are shown in Fig. 2.1.

HA has a disaccharide structure and usually exists as sodium hyaluronate. It is a glycosaminoglycan that has the same structure in animals and bacteria. Therefore, massive amount of HA manufactured from bacteria is harmless to human beings. That is why there is so many HA filler in the market.

Healthy human HA has a molecular weight of 5,000,000–10,000,000 Da; animal-based HA has a molecular weight of 4,000,000–6,000,000 Da, while the molecular weight of bacterial-based HA is 1,500,000–2,500,000 Da. However, the HA filler is made by cross-linking of these HA molecules to form a gel structure; therefore, the molecular weight does not differ much.

2.1 Hyaluronic Acid

HA is a disaccharide present in the skin, synovial fluid, and vitreous humor. Of the 12 g of HA present in a human being, 3 g is dissolved

2.2 HA Filler

HA differs from HA filler. HA is sold in the amorphous form in the market. Since hyaluronidase naturally exists in the human body,

Fig. 2.1 Molecular structure of hyaluronic acid

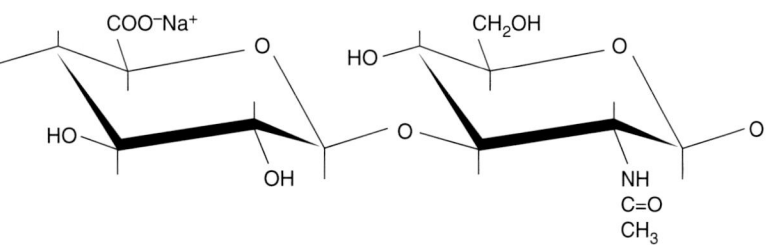

Na glucuronate   N-acetylglucosamine

HA should be cross-linked using a cross-linker to ensure its stability (Fig. 2.2).

1,4-Butanediol diglycidyl ether (BDDE) is a popular cross-linker. Filler properties depend on factors like amount of BDDE used, time to react with BDDE, and reaction temperatures (Fig. 2.3).

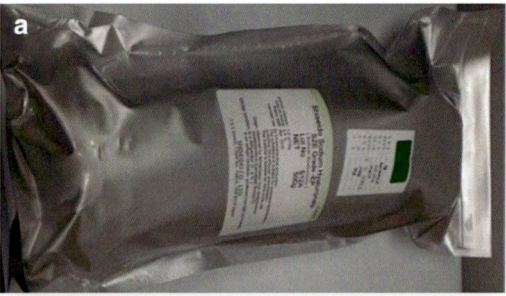

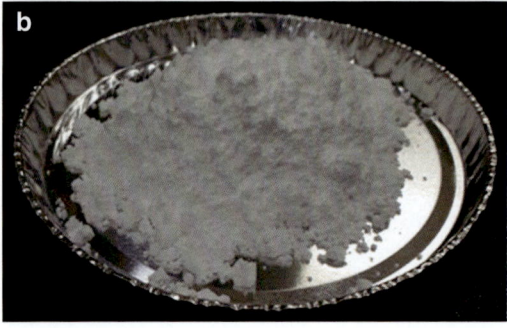

Fig. 2.2 Raw hyaluronic acid. (**a**) Hyaluronic acid product. (**b**) Hyaluronic acid powder

2.3　HA Filler Manufacturing Process

HA filler is made by mixing raw HA powder with a cross-linker, and each company uses different raw products, cross-linker concentrations, reaction times, temperature, and manufacturing process (Fig. 2.4).

Each manufacturer follows a different process. For example, some products are made by reaction at 50 °C for 2–3 hours, while other products are manufactured at 45 °C with a reaction time of 4 hours [1]. The washing process is different for the products subjected to dialysis or those whose manufacture process involves a dehydration and reswelling process. Some products are mixed with non-cross-linked HA at the final stage (Fig. 2.5).

A notable process is the degradation of raw HA by NaOH. At pH <8.0, the molecular structure of the HA carboxyl chain (-COOH) is altered since an ester bond may be formed; at pH >10.0 HA, the hydroxyl chain (-OH) may be involved in the formation of an ether linkage. This ether bond should be linked to BDDE, and a strong bond should be formed. However, since NaOH is alkaline, it may be harmful for the human body; thus, all surfaces should be washed after handling. Unlinked BDDE should also be washed out completely after the reaction [2]. Thus, the washing process is extremely important.

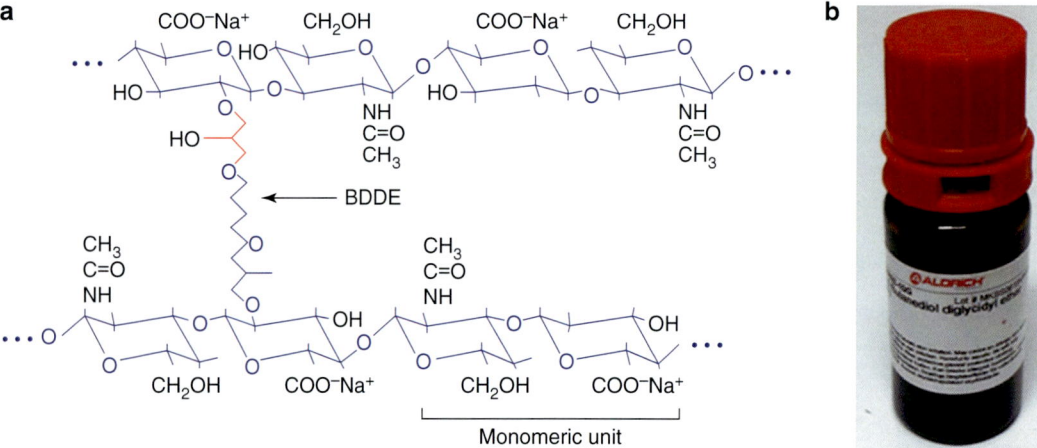

Fig. 2.3 Cross-linking process and cross-linker. (**a**) Molecular structure of the cross-linker. (**b**) Cross-linker: 1,4-butanediol diglycidyl ether (BDDE)

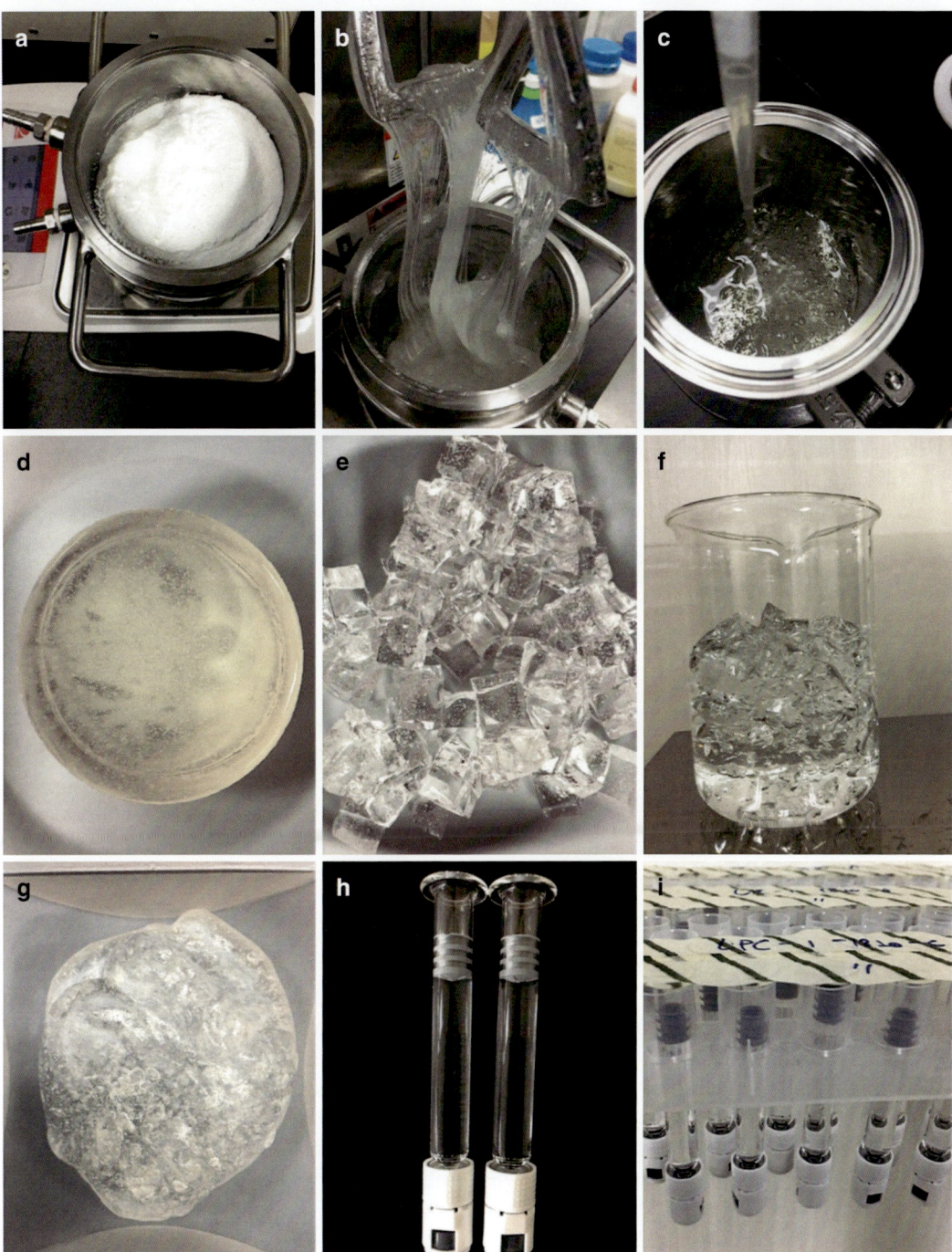

Fig. 2.4 Manufacturing process. (**a**) Weight: weight raw hyaluronic acid. (**b**) Dissolve in NaOH. (**c**) Reaction: mix with 1,4-butanediol diglycidyl ether at appropriate times and temperatures. (**d**) Gel after reaction. (**e**) Cutting: cut the gel to appropriate size. (**f**) Washing: wash off remaining NaOH, free 1,4-butanediol diglycidyl ether, and hyaluronic impurities. (**g**) Sieving: sieve for the appropriate size. (**h**) Filling: fill the syringe. (**i**) Autoclave

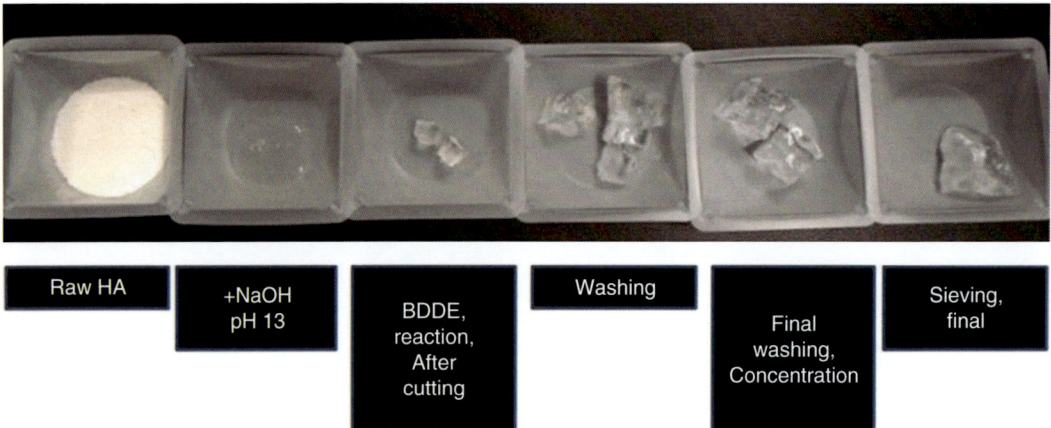

| Raw HA | +NaOH pH 13 | BDDE, reaction, After cutting | Washing | Final washing, Concentration | Sieving, final |

Fig. 2.5 Hyaluronic acid filler change during the manufacturing process

The problem is that BDDE cannot be removed during the washing process. This could be a cause of chronic inflammation. We will discuss these points in Chap. 3, which details filler- induced hypersensitivity inflammation and filler granuloma.

2.4   Properties of HA Fillers

There are hundreds of filler products in the market, each of which has a different manufacturing process, resulting in different properties of the fillers.

2.4.1   Biphasic Versus Monophasic

"Biphasic" and "monophasic" have been used frequently to differentiate among HA fillers. However, this categorization is based on misinterpretations of the term "phase" since it refers to differences among manufacturing processes. However, there are definite differences between Restylane, the most popular biphasic filler, and Juvederm, the most common monophasic filler. Biphasic fillers are known for their relatively high G′ (storage modulus) due to the HA particles within them. On the contrary, monophasic fillers have a relatively low G′ but higher cohesiveness. Between two fillers with the same cohesiveness, the stronger one with a higher G′ is used for nose or chin augmentations. However, products with

a high G′ should have enough cohesiveness to hold the particles together to prevent migration. In contrast, since monophasic fillers have relatively high degrees of cohesiveness, they should be used in wide areas, such as the forehead. Manufacturers are now attempting to make fillers that have the advantages of both monophasic and biphasic fillers.

The author tested 41 products with a rheometer (Tables 2.1 and 2.2).

2.4.2   HA Concentration

Every filler has a declared HA concentration, the content of HA within 1 mL of filler. A product that contains 20 mg of HA is expressed as 20 mg/ mL; when there is a higher amount of HA, the filler would be long lasting and hard. However, since HA is likely to absorb surrounding water molecules, swelling might occur when the equilibrium is broken. Generally, 5.5 mg of HA in 1 mL of water reaches equilibrium, but since HA is cross-linked, there is no strict concentration.

*Differences in the degree of swelling between the HA fillers.

HA is a naturally existing disaccharide in the human body and can pull large amount of water from adjacent tissues. Thus, equilibrium is important to preventing swelling. It is known that 5.5 mg HA in 1 mL reaches equilibrium [3], the solubility of HA in water is 5.5 mg/mL, but the

Table 2.1 Tested biphasic fillers

Product	Restylane	Neobelle	Hyafilia	Cleviel	Yvoire	Cutegel
Company	Galderma (Sweden)	Ildong Aesthetics (Korea)	CHA Meditech (Korea)	Aestura (Korea)	LG chemical (Korea)	BNC (Korea)
Superficial dermis		Skin	Petit			
Dermis	Restylane	Basic		Prime	Classic	
Deep dermis	Perlane	Edge	Classic	Contour	Volume	
Subcutaneous	Restylane SubQ	Contour	Grand		Contour	Cutegel max

Table 2.2 Tested monophasic fillers

Product	Juvederm	E.p.t.q.	Danae	Bellast	Elravie	Neuramis	Chaeum
Company	Allergan (USA)	Jetema (Korea)	CGBio (Korea)	Dongkuk (Korea)	Humedics (Korea)	Medytox (Korea)	Acros (Korea)
Superficial dermis				Vital		Light	
Dermis	Volbella	S100	Original	Soft	Light	Neuramis	No. 1
Deep dermis	Volift	S300	Line	SoftL	Deep	Deep	No. 2
Subcutaneous	Voluma	S500	Contour	Plus, Volume	Ultravolume	Volume	No. 3, No. 4

most common cross-linker BDDE cannot provide a filler of sufficient hardness for lifting capacity. For this reason, the manufacturers make concentrations of 15 mg, 20 mg, 24 mg, and 33 mg; high concentrations would lead to initial swelling. Another cross-linker, divinyl sulfone, can provide sufficient hardness at low concentrations, but it is toxic and rarely used anymore.

2.4.3   Particle Size

When an HA filler contains small particles, it is best used in the dermal layer; in contrast, when it contains larger particles, it is best injected into the subcutaneous layer or beneath. Biphasic filler use is categorized by particle size. Every HA filler can be evaluated by a particle size analyzer that can estimate where it should be used (Fig. 2.6).

2.4.4   Injection Force, Extrusion Force

Injection force is a parameter of how smooth the filler is injected. When the injection force (N) is high, relatively high power is needed to inject them; therefore, every fillers should be tested by needles with standard diameter (Fig. 2.7). The company should specify that the product is easy to inject; therefore, they tend to use a larger-diameter needle during testing. Thus, it is important to record the doctor's own impressions instead of relying on just the company's data.

The graph line shows an abrupt increase followed by a plateau, indicative of filler viscosity. The highest point is called the yield point, at which we can experience abrupt shooting and might yield an unpleasant result or a higher possibility of vascular compromise.

This phenomenon might occur in biphasic filler because of the presence of uneven particles. Thus, the authors recommend the use of a 1–2G larger-diameter needle than that recommended by the filler company.

When a small-diameter needle or cannula is used, the injection force should be high, but a high pressure can cause serious vascular compromises. Needle diameters are compared in Table 2.3.

The author tested injection forces with different diameter needles (Table 2.4).

a

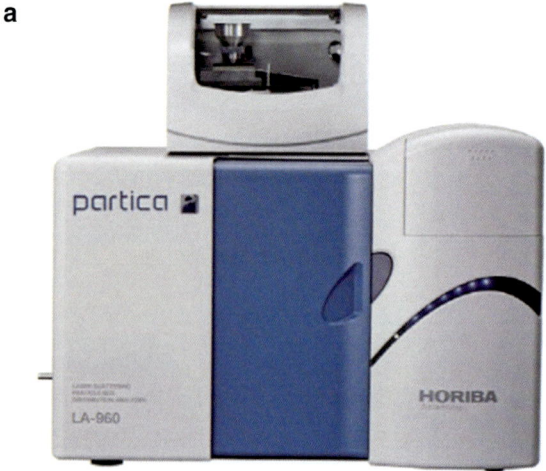

b

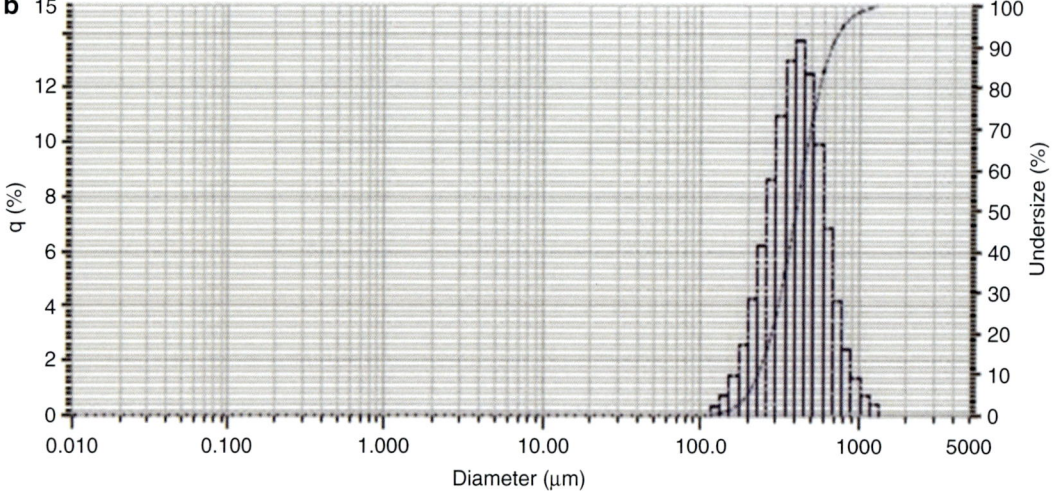

Fig. 2.6 Particle size analyzer results. (**a**) Particle size analyzer. (**b**) Hyaluronic acid filler: average size, 432 μm

Using a small- versus large-diameter needle remains controversial. When using a small-diameter needle, there is a small chance of vessel puncture inside the vessel that can cause an embolism that moves to a farther location. When using a large-diameter needle, there is a greater chance of vessel compromise, but it is impossible to locate inside the vessel, so the pressure is distributed, and emboli cannot move to a farther location (Fig. 2.8).

This fact is very important for blindness or cerebral infarction caused by arterial regurgitation. There are some predisposing factors for blindness, including (1) the needle end should be located inside the artery; (2) the internal carotid artery branch should be used; (3) the injection pressure should be higher than the arterial pressure for arterial regurgitation; and (4) the filler amount should be greater than the arterial volume to cover the central retinal artery.

The use of a small-diameter needle is affected by factors 1 and 3 listed above. As described in Fig. 2.8, a small-diameter needle can enter the artery, and its pressure should be higher; for these reasons, we eliminated two predisposing factors by using a larger-diameter needle.

Fig. 2.7 Injection force
machine and result

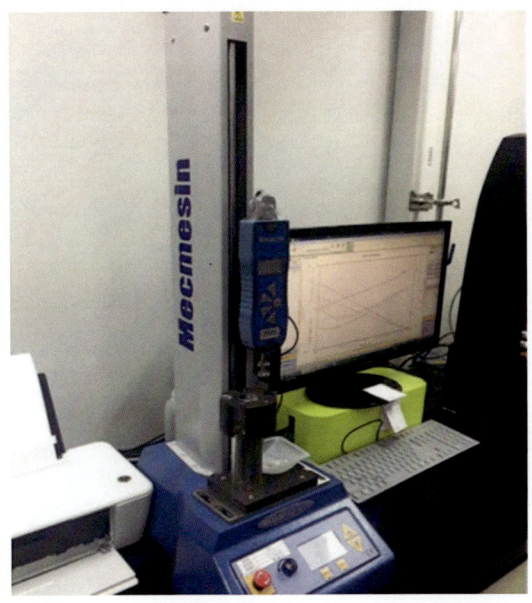

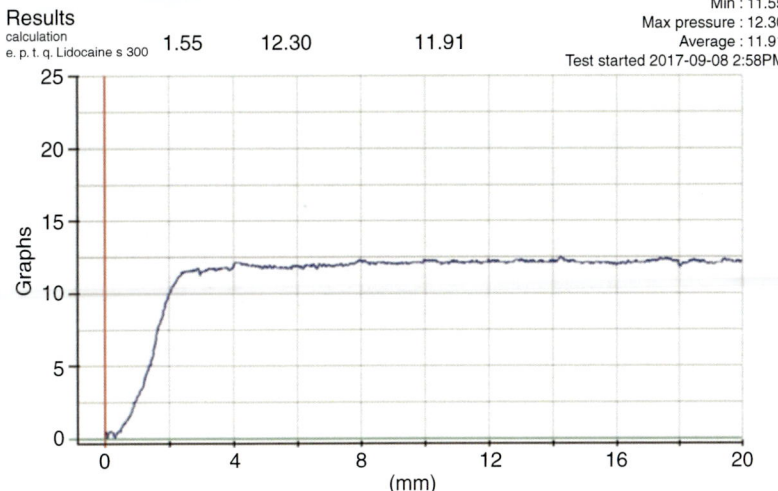

Table 2.3 Needle diameters

	Outer diameter (mm)	Inner diameter (mm)
18G	1.27	0.84
19.5G	0.99	0.69
21G	0.82	0.51
22G	0.71	0.41
23G	0.64	0.34
25G	0.51	0.26
27G	0.41	0.21
29G	0.34	0.18
30G	0.31	0.16

Table 2.4 Injection forces with different diameter needles

	25G	27G	30G
Eptq s50 lidocaine	8.71 N	13.96 N	25.41 N
Eptq s100 lidocaine	9.56 N	13.69 N	26.84 N
Eptq s300 lidocaine	9.5 N	12.8 N	24.29 N
Eptq s500 lidocaine	8.29 N	11.14 N	33.20 N

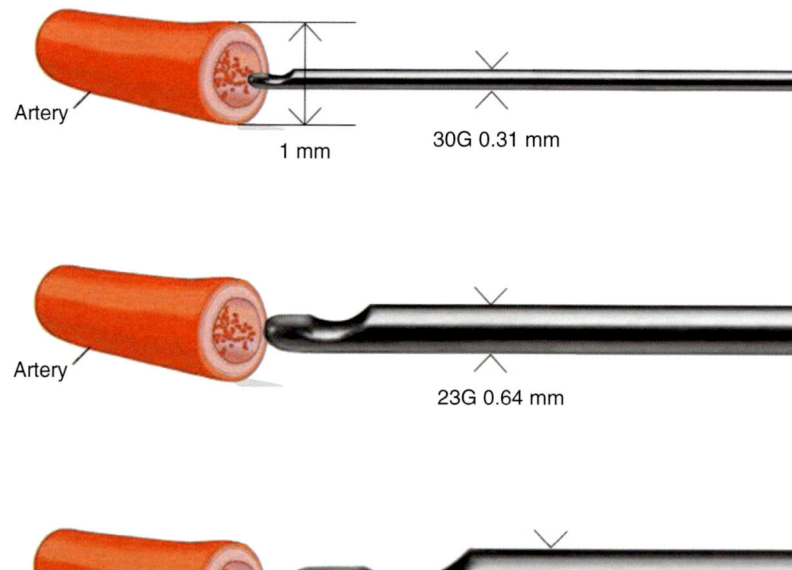

Fig. 2.8 Arterial diameter compared to cannula diameter. Mean diameter of supratrochlear, supraorbital, and dorsal nasal artery is 1 mm

2.4.5 Cross-Linking Ratio, Degree of Modification (MOD)

As described previously, cross-linked HA filler consists of HA and BDDE. The use of a larger amount of BDDE in the manufacturing process can provide long lasting harder fillers. Thus, cross-linking ideally connects the bilateral sides of HA. However, there are some pendent types in which the cross-linker is attached to only one side of the HA. Also called the dangling type, it is useless for HA fillers (Fig. 2.9).

Degree of modification, a parameter of both cross-linked and pendent HA, can be calculated by nuclear magnetic resonance (NMR). However, since MOD consists of both molecules, we should detect each separately. Each molecules can be detected by size exclusion chromatography combined with mass spectrometry (SEC-MS). This machine can be used to separately calculate cross-linked MOD (cMOD) and pendent MOD (pMOD). Thus, in cases of high MOD and high pMOD, the filler does not contain large amounts of cross-linked HA, while many complications might occur due to pendent HA. For example, Restylane has a relatively low reported MOD

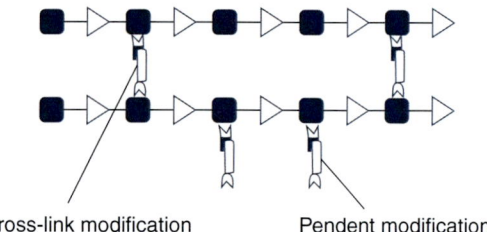

Fig. 2.9 Pendent type BDDE

of 0.8 but has a similar cMOD to those of other products, showing that it is a relatively low pendent type [4]. Recently, the pendent type has been one of the potent possible causes of filler-induced hypersensitivity, so many investigators are analyzing the use of NMR and SEC-MS.

2.4.6 Rheology

Rheology is an objective method to evaluate filler properties. Rheology is also the study of the flow such as viscosity, elasticity, plasticity, thixotropy, and cohesiveness. Filler rheology elasticity and viscosity and cohesiveness are quite important and will be discussed later. Plasticity refers to the propensity of a solid material to undergo permanent deformation under a load, i.e., stress over elasticity. Thixotropy is the property exhibited by certain compounds that are liquid or have low viscosity when agitated or stirred but set slightly when standing still. For example, filler should be in the gel state in the syringe, become a liquid when injected through a needle, and assume a solid state inside human beings. Unfortunately, fillers remain in the liquid state after injection.

Various stresses are applied in humans when filler is injected; using a rheometer, we can estimate filler properties (Figs. 2.10 and 2.11).

These are the relative important parameters of filler rheology:

- G′: Elastic modulus, storage modulus, resistance to deformation

The filler deformation parameter is affected by external stress; when G′ is high, low deformation occurs. This is not an exact parameter of hardness but is closely related. Fillers with higher G′ values will recover their shape better. Biphasic fillers usually have a relatively high G′.

- G″: Viscous modulus, loss modulus

The parameter of filler dissipated energy during shear stress due to friction differs from complex viscosity. Fillers with a high G″ tend to lose energy and become liquid.

- Complex viscosity

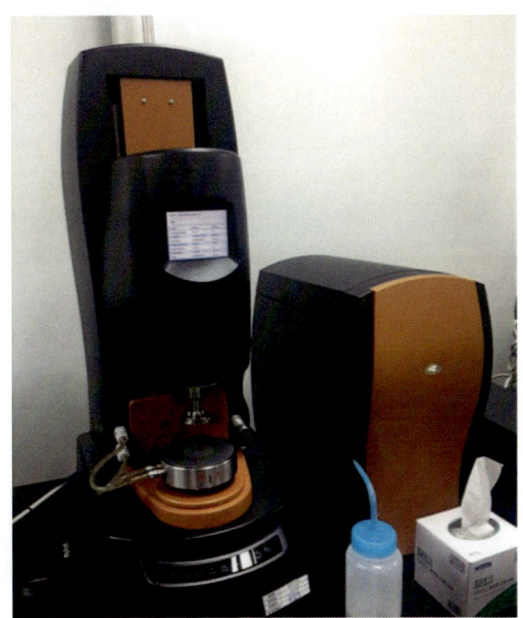

Fig. 2.11   Rheometer

Deformation forces

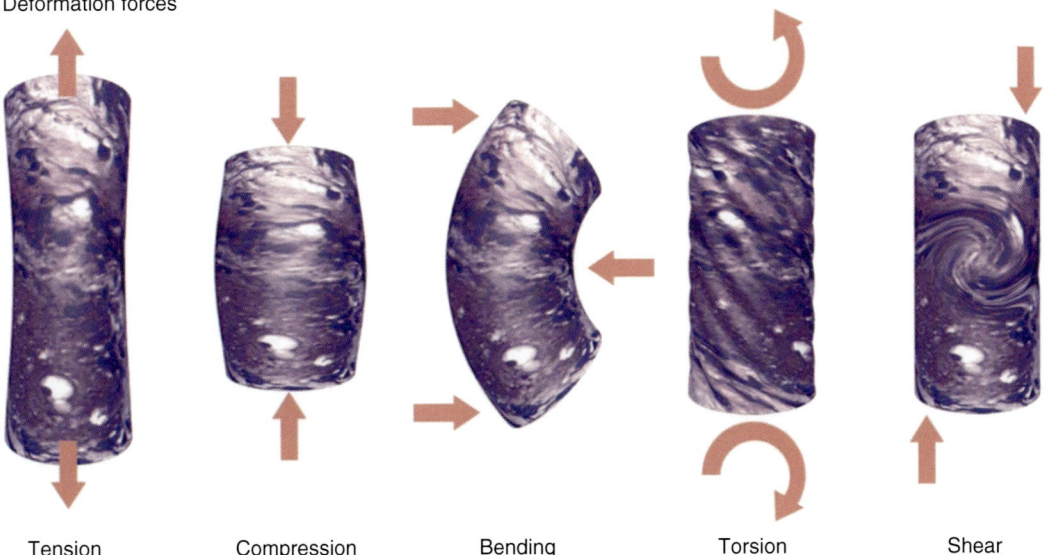

Tension   Compression   Bending   Torsion   Shear

Fig. 2.10   Various stresses placed on fillers

The parameter of a filler's ability to resist flow indicates the filler's thickness and is very much related to injection force.

- Tan δ: tangent delta

This parameter is calculated as follows: G'/G''. This parameter indicates whether a filler is likely to be solid or liquid. A value of tan δ > 1 indicates that it is likely to be a liquid.

- Phase angle

This parameter involves the transformation of tan δ to an angle. When tan δ = 1, then the phase angle is 90°.

- Elasticity: G*

This parameter of filler hardness is calculated by $100 \times G'/(G' + G'')$. It is a percentage of stored energy divided by total energy. For example, if the filler is soft, total energy might be high, but energy loss is also high, meaning that, after the injection of soft filler into the skin, it will be easily deformed by skin compression and has low elasticity.

The rheometric parameters are not always the same; rather, they vary according to plate size, temperature, and frequency. Thus, a G' of 500 does not specifically mean anything; rather, it is used for comparison only (Figs. 2.12 and 2.13).

The author tested 41 different hyaluronic fillers by a rheometer under the same conditions. Each company has its own guidelines, but the results differ little. For example, one filler should be used in the subcutaneous layer according to the manufacturer, but the rheometer parameters are the same as those of another product used in the subdermal layer (Table 2.5).

2.4.7 Cohesiveness

Cohesiveness is not a proper rheological term, but it is a very important parameter determining the filler properties. Unfortunately, it is not objectively calculated, and multiple methods are

required to obtain objective data. A parameter of rheometer, referred to as tack data, serves as a cohesiveness index or indicator of diffusion capacity when injected into saline. Cohesiveness is important because of filler migration and molding procedures. The injected filler should aggregate each other to resist compressive forces.

Manufacturers recommend that some fillers be used in the subcutaneous layer, but some rheological data shows the filler might migrate when injected into the nose or chin because it has insufficient cohesiveness or storage modulus. Thus, it is important to determine filler properties and decide which one is suitable for use.

2.5 Hyaluronidase

HA fillers are used in >80% of the market because they can be degraded by hyaluronidase in cases of complications. Hyaluronidase is classified depending on whether the enzyme is obtained from animal testicles, leeches, or bacteria; hyaluronidase available in the market is usually made from bacterial components. The product is usually made of ovine or bovine testicle or human recombinant DNA and is used for hypodermoclysis by dissolving normal HA but is also used to dissolve HA fillers (off-label use). Hyaluronidase breaks bonds between N-acetylglucosamine C1 and glucuronic acid C4.

There are more than 20 products in the market; some are amorphous (Liporase®), while others are liquid (Hylex®). The product Vitrase® in the United States is made from ovine testicles and is 200 USP. Hylenex® is a human recombinant DNA product that is made with genetic manipulation of Chinese hamster ovarian cells, and it is 150 USP (Fig. 2.14). Hylenex is available at 150 USP and 200 USP in the United States, and 3–4 bottles are used to treat complications such as skin necrosis. However, in some countries like Korea or China, products at 1500 IU are available, so one bottle might be sufficient for the same treatment. (One International Unit [IU] = 1 USP.)

A skin test is recommended before the use of hyaluronidase. Although very rare, an immuno-

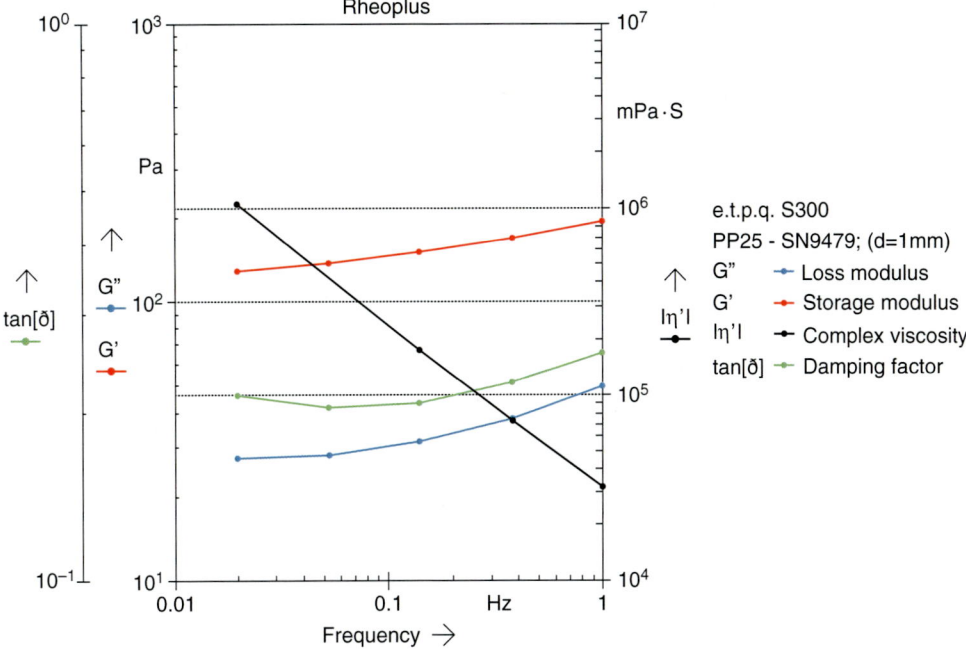

Meas. Pts.	Angular frequency	Storage modulus	Loss modulus	Damping factor	Complex viscosity
	[rad/s]	[Pa]	[Pa]	[1]	[Pa·s]
1	6.28	1.94E+01	5.02E+01	0.258	3.19E+01
2	2.36	1.70E+02	3.89E+01	0.229	7.37E+01
3	0.889	1.52E+02	3.18E+01	0.209	1.75E+02
4	0.334	1.38E+02	2.84E+01	0.205	4.22E+02
5	0.126	1.29E+02	2.76E+01	0.214	1.05E+03

Fig. 2.12 Rheologic result. (Courtesy from Lee et al. [5])

logic reaction can occur since the product is made of animal origin. Its liquid form is also made from animal testicles, and Vitrase® also can induce allergic reactions. Hylenex® might induce an allergic reaction because it contains albumin.

Dose: To dissolve overcorrected or unpleasant results of HA filler injection, the proper dose must be determined. One study described that to dissolve 0.2 mL of Restylane®, 10–30 IU of hyaluronidase is needed, but this is very much dependent on its manufacturing process. Each filler contains different amounts of cross-linking agents and was cross-linked for different amounts of time. An enzyme degradation test is used to calculate the time needed to dissolve HA filler. Every filler has a different degradation time. In the case of 1500 IU hyaluronidase, the use of a very small amount is recommended to dissolve unpleasant results. However, in cases of severe complications such as skin necrosis, a high dose is recommended to completely degrade HA filler. Multiple injections might aggravate pre-damaged skin, and since underdosing can result in leftover filler, an overdose injection is recommended.

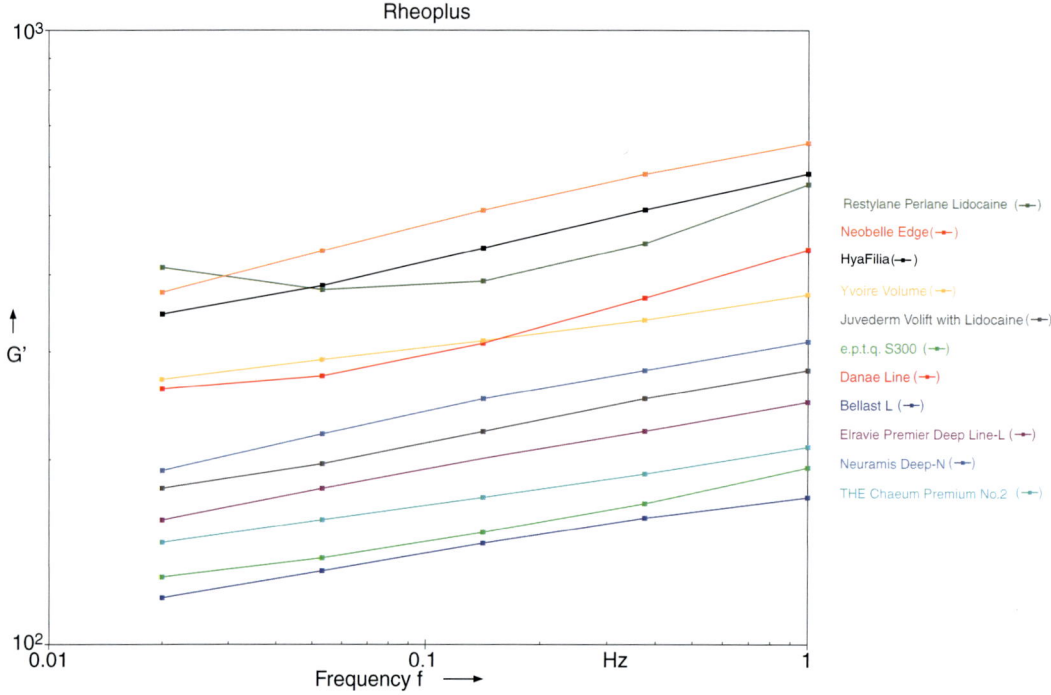

Fig. 2.13 Comparative G′ between multiple fillers (0.02–1 Hz at 25 °C)

Table 2.5 Rheological properties of the fillers

Product	G′ (Pa)	G″ (Pa)	Complex modulus	Tan delta	Complex viscosity (η)	HA conc. (mg/mL)[a]	Cohesiveness (N)	Particle size (μm/mL)	Injection force (N)
Restylane	349	145	378	0.4180	3,011,188	20	0.3509	547 ± 280	8
Perlane	411	199	457	0.4849	3,637,022	20	0.2869	1024 ± 547	16
Restylane SubQ	768	245	806	0.3190	6,420,375	20	0.3387	1393 ± 757	25
Neobelle skin	372	136	396	0.3667	3,157,278	20	1.0296	241 ± 117	12
Neobelle basic	365	116	383	0.3182	3,048,961	20	0.9481	447 ± 215	15
Neobelle edge	374	110	390	0.2936	3,106,528	20	0.9183	941 ± 499	16
Neobelle contour	387	111	403	0.2884	3,207,126	20	0.9019	1472 ± 796	18
Hyafilia petit	247	85	261	0.343	2,080,246	20	0.5536	227 ± 124	10
Hyafilia classic	345	101	359	0.294	2,858,186	20	0.6038	488 ± 267	12
Hyafilia grand	407	166	440	0.407	3,499,743	20	0.5185	991 ± 525	15
Cleviel prime	372	180	413	0.485	3,291,663	33	0.8778	284[b]	16.6
Cleviel contour	857	694	1103	0.81	8,774,267	50	1.536	243[b]	20
Yvoire classic	286	103	304	0.3624	2,424,107	22	0.2894	693 ± 344	9.8
Yvoire volume	253	73	263	0.2910	2,097,766	22	0.3567	1036 ± 581	12.7
Yvoire contour	484	157	509	0.3245	4,049,358	22	0.2867	1258 ± 742	19
Cutegel max	701	286	757	0.41	6,024,716	20	0.57	1106 ± 689[b]	20
Juvederm Volbella	99	21	101	0.2189	814,593	15	0.3046	634 ± 255	8
Juvederm Volift	179	42	184	0.2343	1,468,502	17.5	0.3417	644 ± 303	10

Table 2.5 (continued)

Product	G′ (Pa)	G″ (Pa)	Complex modulus	Tan delta	Complex viscosity (η)	HA conc. (mg/mL)[a]	Cohesiveness (N)	Particle size (μm/mL)	Injection force (N)
Juvederm Voluma	284	58	290	0.2066	2,309,805	20	0.4043	703 ± 389	25
E.p.t.q.S100	37	15	40	0.4269	323,859	24	0.4184	UD	19.6
E.p.t.q.S300	128	27	131	0.2137	1,048,864	24	0.6102	UD	29.4
E.p.t.q.S500	224	57	231	0.2551	1,847,607	24	0.8776	296 ± 168	31
Danae original	154	81	174	0.5279	1,389,716	20	0.5531	646 ± 352	9.8
Danae line	260	100	279	0.3869	2,222,574	20	0.3785	1162 ± 668	19
Danae contour	469	134	488	0.2873	3,887,740	20	0.46	1291 ± 762	37.2
Bellast vital	128	72	147	0.5636	1,170,954	20	0.2362	685 ± 386	15
Bellast soft L	94	22	97	0.2400	775,485	20	0.2285	683 ± 321	12
Bellast L	119	25	122	0.2135	969,817	20	0.2880	684 ± 242	16
Bellast plus	87	18	89	0.2062	714,771	20	0.5093	652 ± 319	32.3
Bellast volume	106	23	108	0.215	866,658	20	0.4458	685 ± 313	33
Elravie premier light	140	34	144	0.2431	1,151,729	23	0.5260	UD	23
Elravie premier deep line	159	39	164	0.2486	1,309,982	23	0.5874	UD	25
Elravie premier ultra volume	198	59	207	0.2985	1,646,177	23	0.8478	UD	24.5
Neuramis light	4	4	6	1.0530	51,271	20	0.2049	322 ± 133	8
Neuramis	57	24	133	0.4284	499,532	20	0.4532	433 ± 178	12.7
Neuramis deep	127	38	133	0.3000	1,061,307	20	0.5998	411 ± 171	16.6
Neuramis volume	281	71	290	0.2551	2,309,230	20	0.8003	402 ± 175	22.5
Chaeum No. 1	76	28	81	0.3733	651,115	24	0.4888	480 ± 204	14.7
Chaeum No. 2	146	29	149	0.2036	1,193,756	20	0.6716	473 ± 242	34.3
Chaeum No. 3	232	52	238	0.2200	1,896,742	20	0.7474	596 ± 291	37.2
Chaeum No. 4	340	68	347	0.2013	2,766,277	20	0.9180	664 ± 348	54.8

SD standard deviation
[a]From the package insert; product information provided by the manufacturer
[b]Median

The author recommends the use of 750 IU to degrade 1 mL of HA filler. This is generally an overdose, but it is important to completely degrade the filler. If not dissolved by this amount, the area assumed to be the filler could actually be a granuloma.

Some patients might ask to dissolve just part of the injected filler, but it is better to dissolve all the filler and reinject new filler. Since it is impossible to control the amount of degraded filler and the remaining amount of filler by injection of hyaluronidase, it is difficult to fulfill this patient's request. When an insufficient dose of hyaluroni-dase is injected, another dose should be injected; if an overdose is injected, the filler should be reinjected.

Allergy: A skin test is recommended but not usually performed before the injection. Most products have the possibility of causing immunologic reactions, and the literature described incidences of urticaria and angioedema of <0.1%. Symptoms are severe swelling in the injected area <2 hours after injection. Thus, patients must be warned of the possibility prior to injection.

Treatments include oral antihistamines and corticosteroids.

Fig. 2.14 Variable hyaluronidase products. (**a**) Vitrase (United States) 200 USP. (**b**) Hylenex (United States) 150 USP. (**c**) Hyalase (South Korea) 1500 IU powder. (**d**) Liporase (South Korea) 1500 IU powder. (**e**) Hylex (South Korea) 1500 IU liquid. (**f**) Shanghai product (China) 1500 IU powder

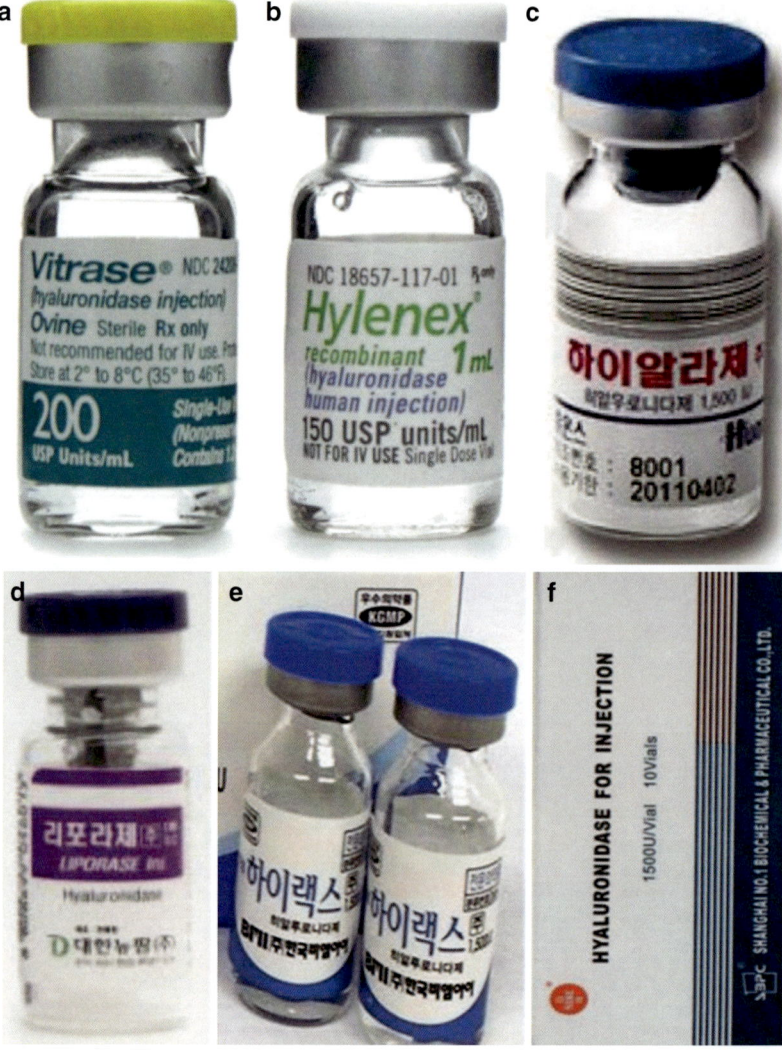

References

1. Choi SC, Yoo MA, Lee SY, Lee HJ, Son DH, Jung J, et al. Modulation of biomechanical properties of hyaluronic acid hydrogels by crosslinking agents. J Biomed Mater Res A. 2015;103(9):3072–80.
2. De Boulle K, Glogau R, Kono T, Nathan M, Tezel A, Roca-Martinez JX, et al. A review of the metabolism of 1,4-butanediol diglycidyl ether-crosslinked hyaluronic acid dermal fillers. Dermatol Surg. 2013;39(12):1758–66.
3. Tezel A, Fredrickson GH. The science of hyaluronic acid dermal fillers. J Cosmet Laser Ther. 2008;10(1):35–42.
4. Yang B, Guo X, Zang H, Liu J. Determination of modification degree in BDDE-modified hyaluronic acid hydrogel by SEC/MS. Carbohydr Polym. 2015;131:233–9.
5. Lee W, Yoon J-H, Koh I-S, Oh W, Kim K-W, Yang E-J. Clinical application of a new hyaluronic acid filler based on its rheological properties and the anatomical site of injection. Biomed Derm. 2018; 2(1):22.

3

Filler-Induced Hypersensitivity Inflammation and Granuloma

Hyaluronic acid filler is retained inside the human body for at least 1 year. Compared to drugs that are absorbed immediately, filler takes a significant amount of time to degrade. During this time, the filler may attack the human immune system and cause serious complications. Therefore, the filler should be manufactured aseptically, and new fillers should be assessed carefully for adverse effects. Many criteria for product licensure depend on laboratory data regarding any unexpected complications of a filler inside the human body.

The most common cause of chronic complications might be filler-induced hypersensitivity inflammation and filler-induced granuloma. Filler-induced hypersensitivity inflammation occurs periodically and manifests as mild swelling to severe edema. This symptom is usually relieved by anti-inflammatory drugs, which are used to treat it. However, repeated hypersensitivity tends to result in filler-induced granuloma, which usually requires surgical treatment. Thus, whenever this kind of symptom occurs, doctors should prevent granuloma formation by removing the filler at an early stage.

3.1 Filler-Induced Hypersensitivity Inflammation

Filler-induced hypersensitivity inflammation is also called repeated tissue reaction, immune reaction, and delayed swelling.

3.1.1 Pathophysiology

Filler-induced hypersensitivity is considered a type IV hypersensitivity. The human immune system treats the filler as an antigen, thus activating macrophages and T lymphocytes to aggregate macrophages in the area of inflammation. This inflammation manifests as swelling and pain 2–3 weeks after the filler injection, and chronic inflammation can lead to granuloma formulation.

The pathophysiology of this phenomenon is not clear; however, multiple suggested causes include filler toxicity, impurities, osmolarity, pH imbalances, and endotoxins. To understand these possible causes, we must study the manufacturing processes as described in Chap. 2.

Hyaluronic acid filler is composed of hyaluronic acid mixed with a crosslinker (usually 1,4-butanediol diglycidyl ether [BDDE]). Multiple possible causes of filler-induced hypersensitivity include:

1. Raw hyaluronic acid: Hyaluronic acid is usually produced from bacterial hyaluronic acid, and large amount of hyaluronic acid power is commonly sold (Chap. 2). Among the bacteria, the *Streptococcus* species are used that may contain bacterial protein, DNA, and endotoxin.
2. Hyaluronic acid is usually dissolved using a highly alkaline solution such as NaOH during the manufacturing process. The disaccharide product hyaluronic acid could be dissolved to

© Springer Nature Singapore Pte Ltd. 2019
I. S. Koh, W. Lee, *Filler Complications*, https://doi.org/10.1007/978-981-13-6639-0_3

a monosaccharide, and its by-product might induce an undesirable reaction in the human body. Moreover, the last step in the manufacturing process, washing, may not eliminate all of the NaOH solution.

3. Crosslinking process: Raw hyaluronic acid is converted to a long-duration hyaluronic acid filler by a crosslinking process using BDDE. The problem is some of this crosslinker links to just one side of the hyaluronic acid, creating a pendant type crosslinker (Fig. 3.1).

When the washing process is properly done, the free and native types are washed out. However, the pendant type remains, making it a highly suspected cause of the filler-induced hypersensitivity reaction. Additionally, by-products as a result of BDDE metabolism could cause some irritation, raising the possibility of human immune reactions (Fig. 3.2).

Even when the products are purchased from the same company, products with a relatively high concentration of hyaluronic acid are associated with a higher incidence of filler-induced hypersensitivity. For this reason, BDDE is an important hypersensitivity-related factor. Cases

in which a large amount of filler is injected or multiple injections are performed show a higher incidence of this complication.

Raw hyaluronic acid is classified based on its usage as ingestion, cosmetic, and medical products; the latter is divided into injection and ophthalmologic products. Generally speaking, when the grade is higher, the cost is higher. Thus, a low-cost product generally has more impurities and induces greater hypersensitivity. Therefore, if the product is low cost, the possible associated complications should be considered.

Possible causes of filler-induced hypersensitivity are shown in Table 3.1.

From the injector's perspective, multiple causes are suspected. The use of a large amount of filler exposes the human body to more foreign bodies and might increase the incidence of hypersensitivity. Multiple injections, a large amount of filler injection, and the use of multiple kinds of products can cause greater hypersensitivity. Injections made into multiple layers can expose more surfaces to foreign bodies and increase the risk of inflammation. Few doctors propose injecting filler using insulin syringes, but this can change the physical properties of fillers and cause greater degrees of inflammation. This method

Fig. 3.1 Various forms of 1,4 butanediol diglycidyl ether. (**a**) Crosslinked. (**b**) Pendant. (**c**) Free. (**d**) Native: final quality test only detects this form (<2 ppm)

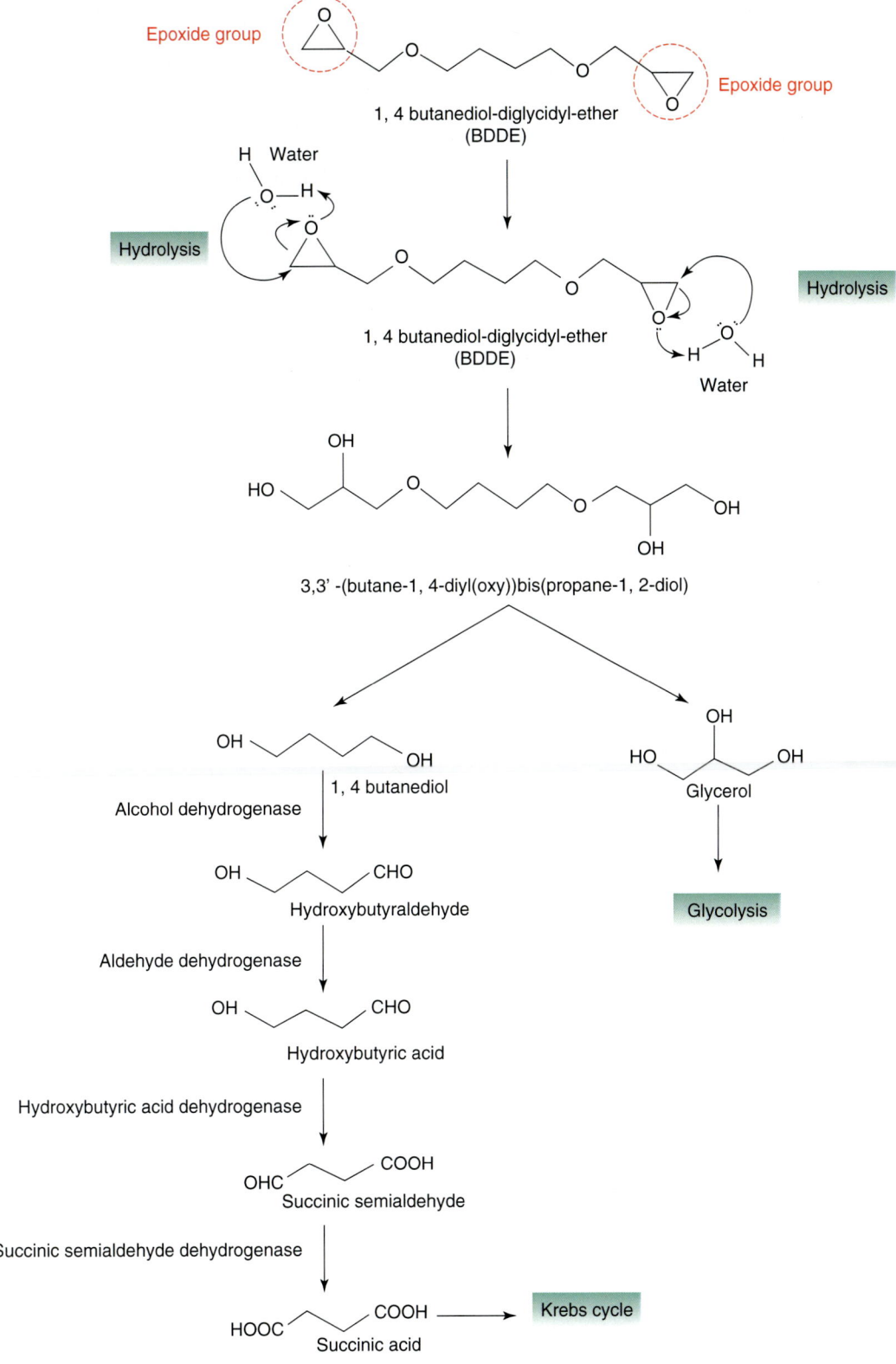

Fig. 3.2 BDDE metabolism. BDDE is dissolved to glycerol and 1,4-butanediol, which is metabolized to hydroxybutyralde-hyde, hydroxybutyric acid, succinic semialdehyde, and finally succinic acid. BDDE, 1,4 butanediol diglycidyl ether

Table 3.1 Possible causes of filler-induced hypersensitivity

Filler	Injector	Patient
Raw material	Injection times	Repetitive stimuli
Impurities	Amount of injection	Personal immunology
Crosslinker	Multiple products	
Additives	Multiple injection area	
Manufacturing process	Contact surfaces	
Hyaluronic acid concentration	Highly molding	
Hyaluronic acid particle size	Exchange syringe	
	Septic procedure	

can also increase the risk of infection. A highly molding procedure is also not advisable.

From the patient's perspective, stimulation should be avoided in the injected area as much as possible. The patient's immunologic state is very important, as a depressed immunologic state, such as the common cold or a highly stressed state, can increase the incidence of hypersensitivity.

3.1.2 Symptoms

Swelling is the most common symptom of a hypersensitivity reaction. More severe symptoms include tenderness, pain, and fever. The symptom presentation starts within 2 weeks after injection as the human body reacts to the foreign body, usually in one region and spreading to adjacent regions.

Symptoms are usually associated with the patient's health status. Common cold, menstrual periods, alcohol intake, and other stresses might decrease the patient's immunologic status and induce swelling. Initially, subclinical swelling and other symptoms that might go unnoticed occur, but the symptoms usually become severe. Clinicians should consider filler-induced hypersensitivity after noting the following symptoms (Table 3.2; Figs. 3.3, 3.4, and 3.5).

The most common sites are the cheek, chin, and premaxillary region, followed by the lip, nose, periocular area, and forehead. Although the cheek, chin, and premaxillary regions receive relatively large amount of fillers, swelling is easily detected in these areas.

3.1.3 Differential Diagnosis

The use of filler injections has increased, and patients tend to complain of various associated symptoms. Thus, it is essential to differentiate between filler-induced hypersensitivity and natural swelling. Filler-induced hypersensitivity tends to develop at least 2 weeks post-injection. They also usually develop unilaterally at the nasojugal groove area and cheek and spread to other locations.

Filler-induced hypersensitivity tends to develop according to a patient's immunologic status, such as during menstrual periods, common cold, or in cases of a depressed immunologic status. Filler-induced hypersensitivity usually develops unilaterally and subsides with anti-inflammatory drug use, whereas false hypersensitivity swelling usually does not subside. When filler-induced hypersensitivity continues, a granuloma develops and multiple nodules are detectable at the lesion. A granuloma can be detected by ultrasound (Table 3.3).

3.1.4 Treatment

Anti-inflammatory drugs are generally effective in cases of mild swelling or tenderness. Steroids can improve symptoms but are not essentially needed. The question is whether symptom improvement cures filler-induced hypersensitivity. Once filler has induced hypersensitivity, it will act as a foreign body antigen, so all hyaluronic acid filler may require elimination by hyaluronidase. The best timing for hyaluronidase administration is when the hypersensitivity first occurs, but it is not easy to convince the patient of the need to dissolve the filler. Thus, it is recommended that the clinician tells the patient about possible recurrence of hypersensitivity and the need to dissolve the fillers.

When dissolving the filler, it is recommended that all fillers be injected at the same time. If only part of the filler is dissolved, the remnant filler might induce another hypersensitivity reaction.

The dosage of the dissolving compound should be higher than the dosage of the filler to ensure dissolution of all the fillers. We prefer to use half a bottle at once (750 IU). This is generally a high dose, but the dosage should be enough to dissolve the filler; if the filler does not dissolve, it might not be hyaluronic acid.

When symptoms recur even after hyaluronidase injection, the clinician should check the granuloma or nodule using an ultrasound device and inject a higher dose of hyaluronidase. When symptoms recur after the second hyaluronidase injection, computed tomography or magnetic resonance imaging should be used to detect occult granuloma and/or the patient should be transferred to special filler complication clinics.

Table 3.2 Symptoms of filler-induced hypersensitivity

Symptoms	Swelling 2 weeks after injection
	Repetitive swelling according to patient's health status
	Spreading pattern of swelling
	Swelling subsides with anti-inflammatory drug administration

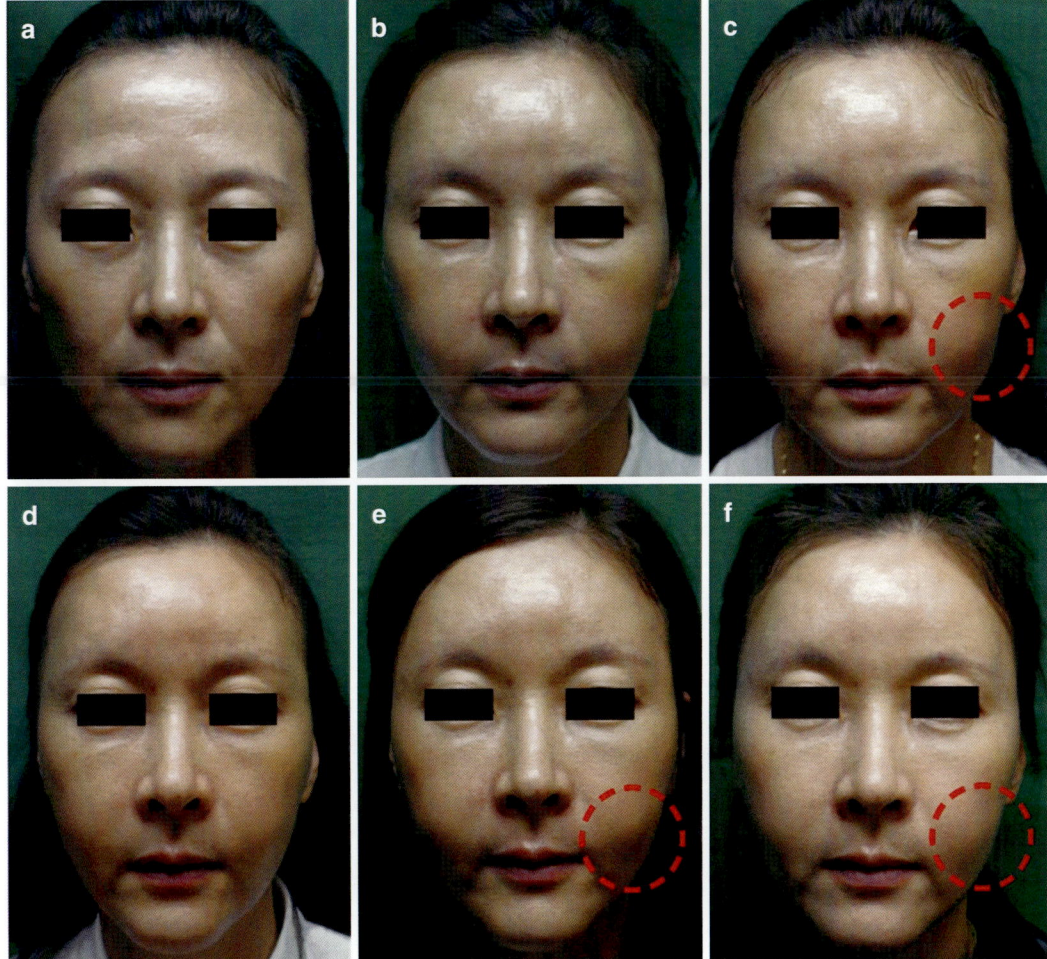

Fig. 3.3 Filler-induced hypersensitivity after the injection of the hyaluronic acid filler. (**a**) Before injection. (**b**) Twelve days post-injection into the cheek, nasojugal groove, nasolabial fold, forehead, and temple. (**c**) Left cheek swelling at 14 days post-injection. (**d**) Symptoms subsided 18 days post-injection. (**e**) Repetitive swelling occurred 25 days post-injection. (**f**) Repetitive swelling occurred 71 days post-injection

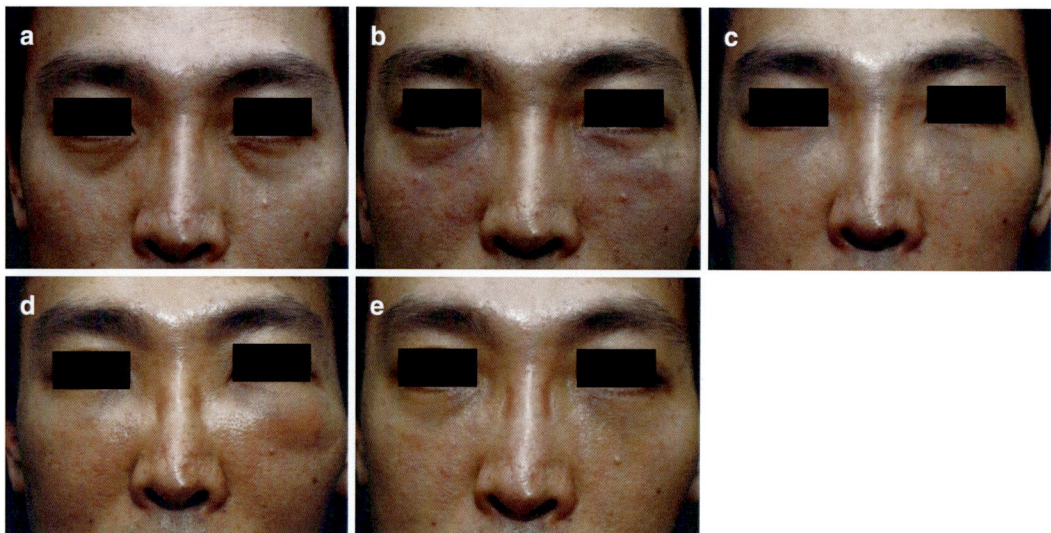

Fig. 3.4 Filler-induced hypersensitivity after injection of the hyaluronic acid filler. (**a**) Preinjection. (**b**) Tear trough correction immediately after injection. (**c**) One week post-injection. (**d**) Severe swelling 10 days post-injection treated by hyaluronidase. (**e**) Swelling subsided 5 days post-injection

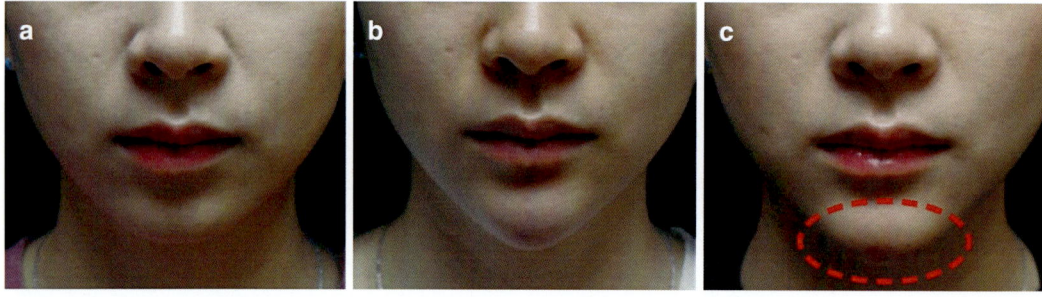

Fig. 3.5 Filler-induced hypersensitivity and granuloma after injection of the hyaluronic acid filler. (**a**) Preinjection. (**b**) One day post-injection. (**c**) Repetitive swelling and granuloma development at 3 days post-injection

Table 3.3 Differential diagnosis

	Filler-induced hypersensitivity	Swelling
Onset	>2 weeks post-injection	Immediate or <2 weeks post-injection
Location	Usually unilateral	Usually in the full face
Pattern	Intermittently	Continuous
Patient's immune status	Menstrual period, common cold, stress	Not related
Severity	Facial asymmetry	Minimal
Nodularity	Hard multiple irregular nodules	Smooth contour
Anti-inflammatory drug	Symptoms subside	Less effective

3.2 Filler Granuloma

The incidence of filler-induced granuloma has increased recently; therefore, precise diagnosis and treatment are required.

3.2.1 Pathophysiology

Repetitive filler-induced hypersensitivity inflammation would induce a granuloma. Repetitive inflammation causes a filler capsule of increasing size. The filler is recognized as a foreign body that induces inflammation and hypersensitivity. Macrophages emerge to phagocytize foreign bodies but fail and then develop into multinucleated giant cells. Fibroblasts are activated by the macrophages, and a fibrous capsule develops as a hard lump. This inflammatory process is worsened by any infection, presence of biofilm, and impaired immunologic status.

A granuloma develops by this process over a period of at least 3 months. A small nodule develops prior to a hard, tender granuloma (Fig. 3.6); thereafter, an irregular and hard granuloma is formed.

A granuloma can be located at the nose, forehead, anterior malar area, cheek, chin, and lips and is related to the incidence of filler injection and closely related to filler-induced hypersensitivity.

The first symptom is a nodule, so it is helpful to diagnose granuloma by accurate history taking and ultrasonography.

A granuloma can also be induced by the use of fillers such as polyacrylamide gel or foreign body products such as silicone.

final shape. A cystic-type granuloma is usually induced by hyaluronic acid filler or hyaluronic acid filler located at a cyst. A nodular-type granuloma usually contains multiple nodules and is induced by hyaluronic acid filler or particle fillers such as calcium hydroxyapatite filler, polycaprolactone filler, and polylactic acid filler.

A sclerosing-type granuloma is usually seen after the injection of the polymethyl methacrylate filler or a foreign body filler such as silicone gel or paraffin. This type of granuloma can also be seen after a long-term infection or hypersensitivity induced by a hyaluronic acid filler injection. It can also be seen after the inappropriate repetitive treatment of a previous granuloma.

An infiltrating-type granuloma manifests as a huge lump with swelling that consists of filler and inflammatory cells. It usually develops after exposure to foreign bodies or permanent fillers (Figs. 3.7, 3.8, 3.9, 3.10, 3.11, 3.12, and 3.13).

3.2.2   Classifications

Granulomas can be classified as cystic, nodular, sclerosing, or infiltrating depending on their

3.2.3   Treatments

Multiple treatments are proposed. Firstly, hyaluronidase after hyaluronic acid filler is injected.

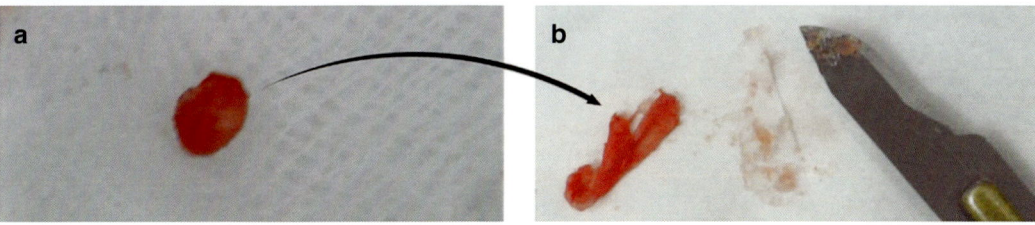

Fig. 3.6 Filler-induced granuloma after injection of the hyaluronic acid filler. Two years after injection of the hyaluronic acid filler. (**a**) Capsular lump. (**b**) Hyaluronic acid filler present inside the capsule

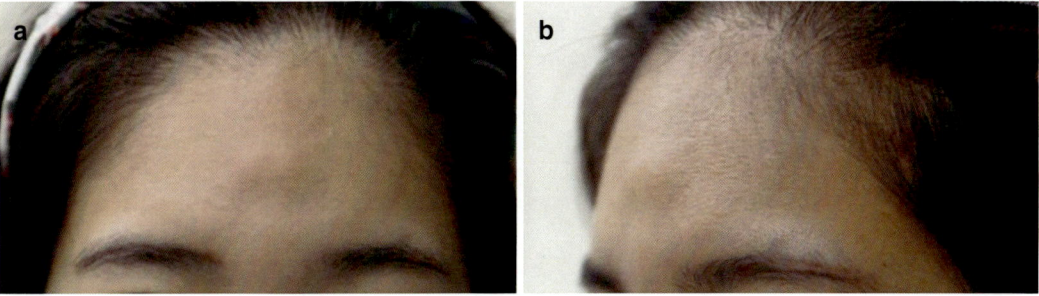

Fig. 3.7 Cystic-type granuloma 2 years after the injection of hyaluronic acid filler. (**a**) Cystic-type granuloma in the center of the forehead. (**b**) Three-quarter view

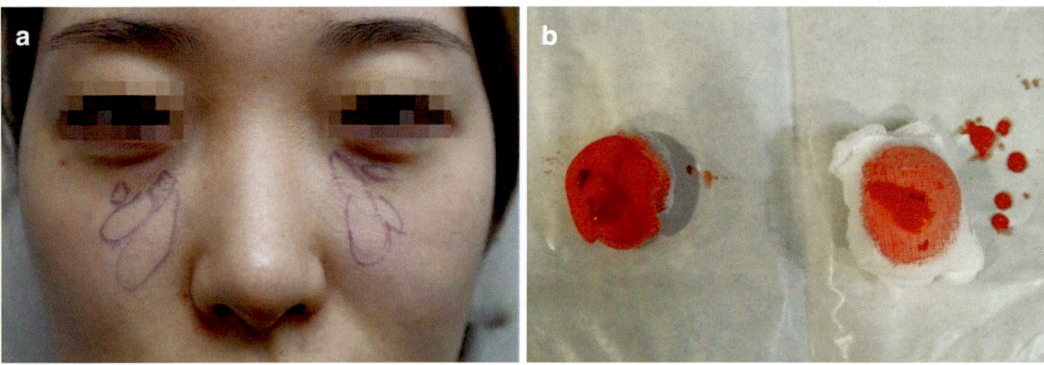

Fig. 3.8 Cystic-type granuloma 1 year after injection of the hyaluronic acid filler. (**a**) Preoperative design. (**b**) Granuloma after negative pressure suction removal

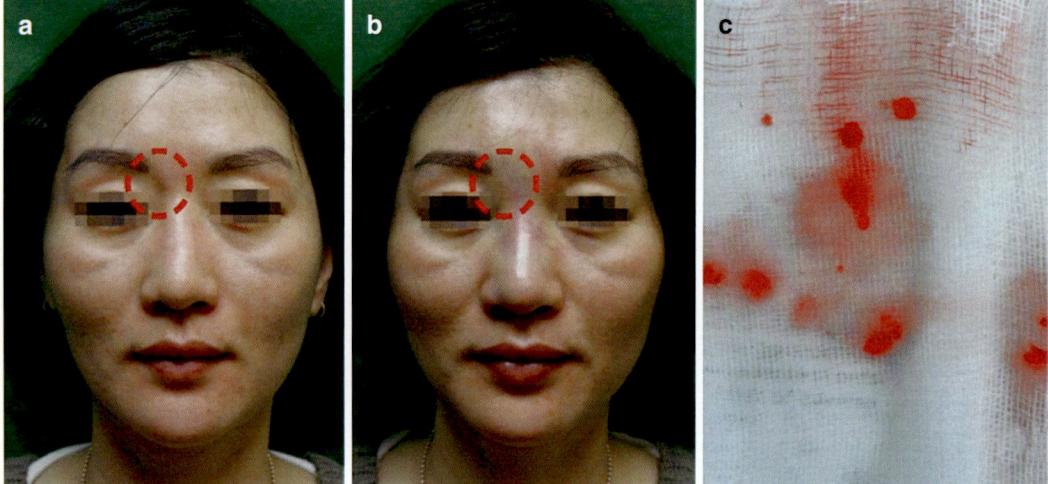

Fig. 3.9 Cystic-type granuloma after injection of the hyaluronic acid filler. Granuloma followed by repetitive filler-induced hypersensitivity after removal of the hyaluronic acid filler using negative pressure suction. (**a**) Cystic-type granuloma at the nasal root. (**b**) View immediate after negative pressure suction removal. (**c**) Granuloma removed by negative pressure suction

Hyaluronidase should be injected into the capsule of a cyst or nodule, usually at a high dose (1500 IU of hyaluronidase mixed with 2 mL of normal saline). However, a granuloma is rarely completely treated by hyaluronidase injection alone since it likely exists as multiple rather than a single capsule. Thus, removal of the filler as well as surgical removal of the capsule is recommended. Surgical excision is the best method to remove all of the fillers and capsules, but surgical

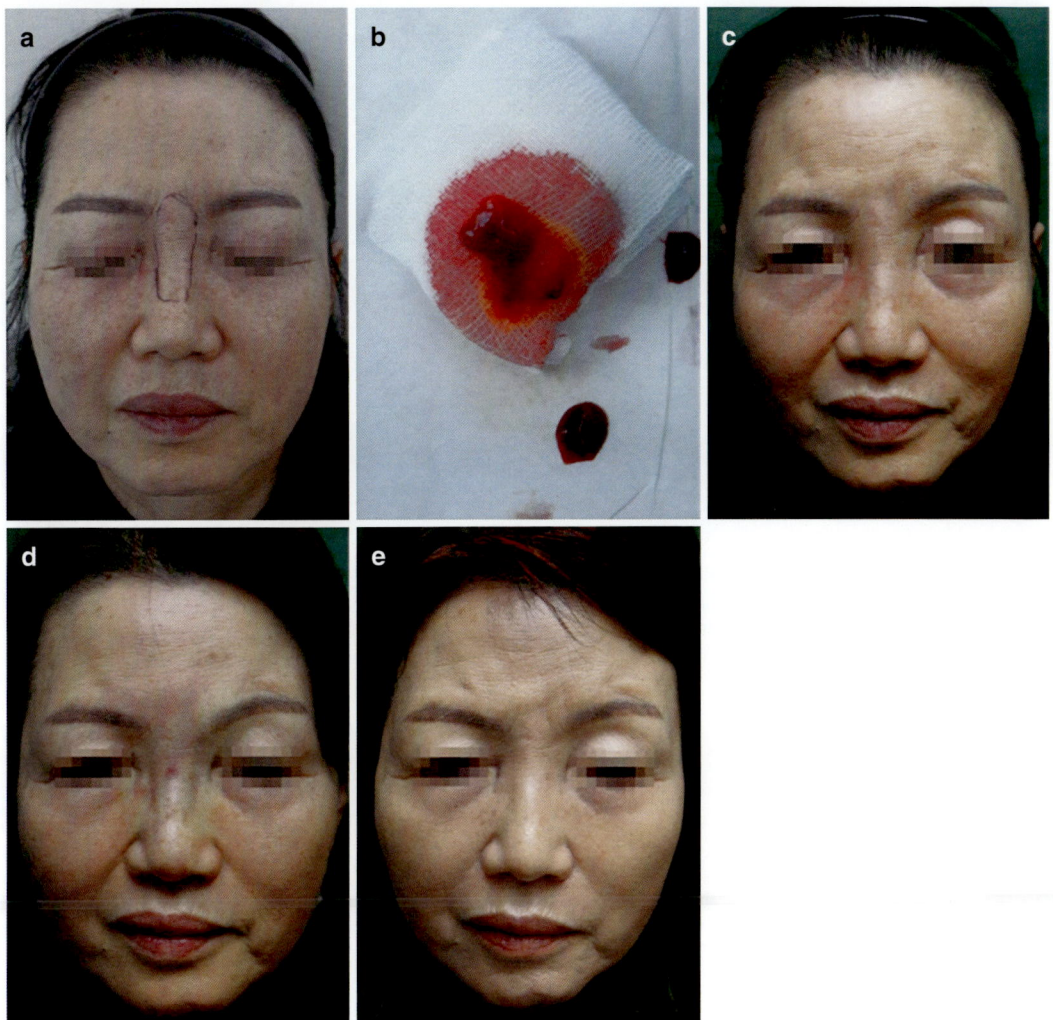

Fig. 3.10 Nodular-type granuloma 6 years after injection of the permanent filler. (**a**) Preoperative design. (**b**) Granuloma removed by negative suction. (**c**) Preoperative view. (**d**) View immediate postoperative. (**e**) View 7 months postoperative

sequelae such as scarring and depressive wounds can develop, for which we prefer to employ negative pressure suction.

Laser-assisted dissolving can be useful, but the best method is the surgeon palpating the granuloma during negative pressure suction.

A steroid injection is sometimes performed, but it can cause the development of depressive wounds. When using hyaluronidase, the use of two or three injections is recommended; if there is no response, a surgical procedure should be performed.

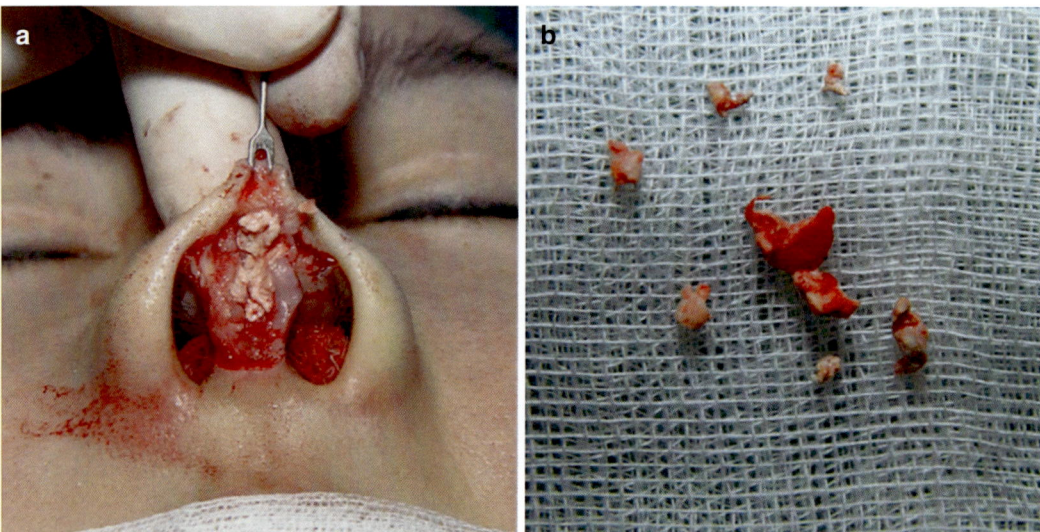

Fig. 3.11 Nodular-type granuloma after injection of the calcium hydroxyapatite filler. Nodular-type granuloma induced by calcium particles after absorption of the carrier gel of calcium hydroxyapatite filler. (**a**) Nodular-type granuloma induced by calcium particles at 6 months after the injection of calcium hydroxyapatite filler. (**b**) Removed calcium hydroxyapatite filler-induced granuloma

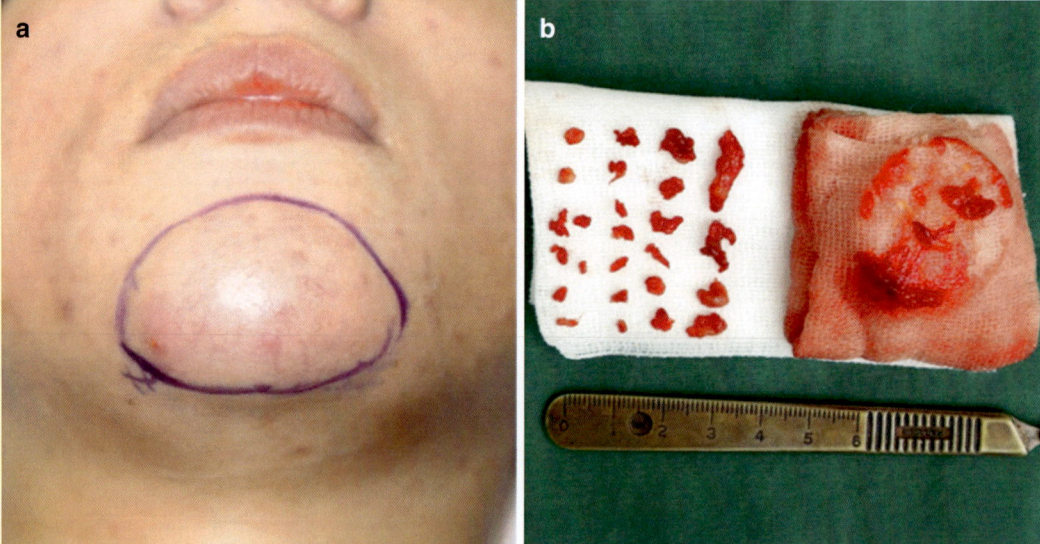

Fig. 3.12 Sclerosing-type granuloma after injection of the permanent polymethyl methacrylate filler into the chin. (**a**) Preoperative design. (**b**) Sclerosing-type granuloma removed by negative pressure suction

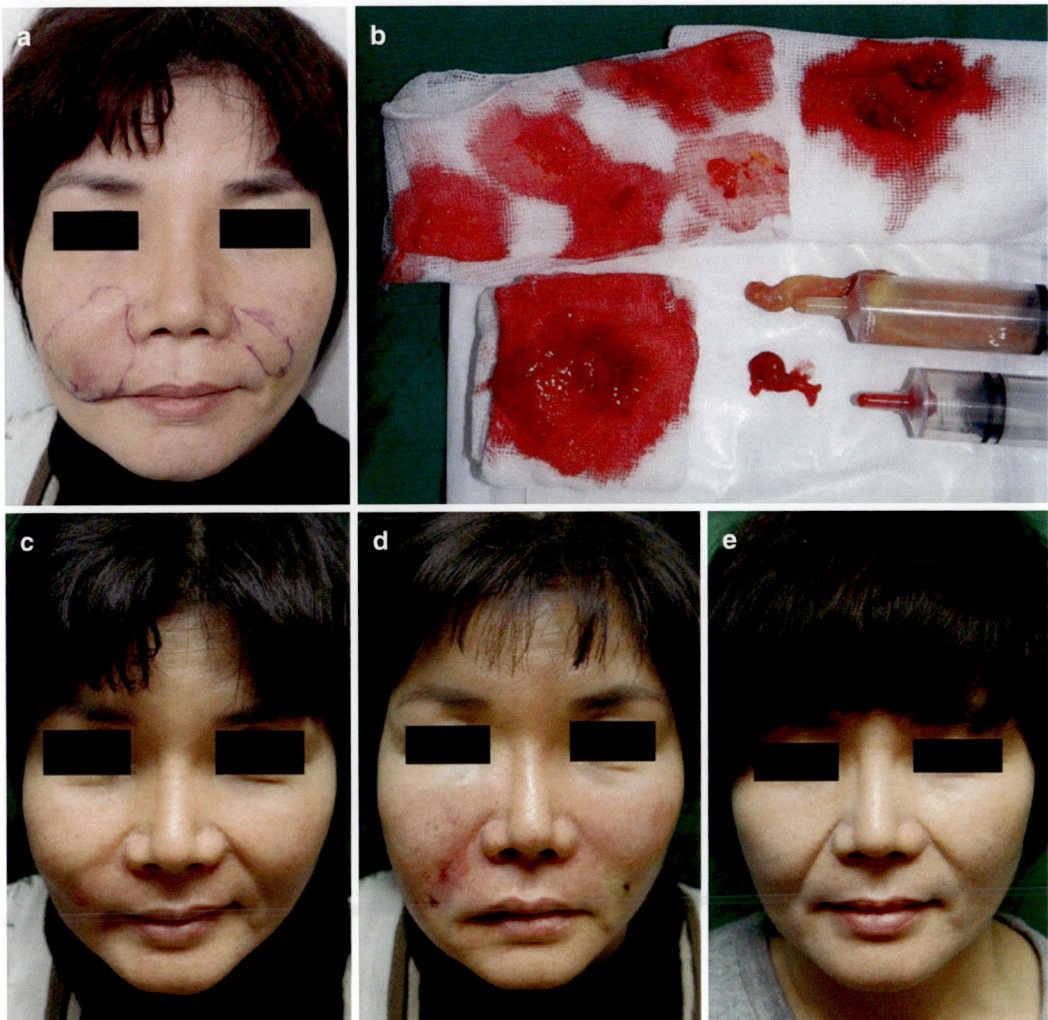

Fig. 3.13 Infiltrating-type granuloma 6 years after injection of the permanent filler. (**a**) Preoperative design. (**b**) Infiltrating-type granuloma removed by negative pressure suction. Permanent filler and inflammatory cells are visible. (**c**) Preoperative view. (**d**) View immediately postoperative. (**e**) View at 2 months postoperative

Further Reading

1. Bhojani-Lynch T. Late-onset inflammatory response to hyaluronic acid dermal fillers. Plast Reconstr Surg Glob Open. 2017;5(12):e1532.
2. De Boulle K, Glogau R, Kono T, Nathan M, Tezel A, Roca-Martinez JX, et al. A review of the metabolism of 1,4-butanediol diglycidyl ether-crosslinked hyaluronic acid dermal fillers. Dermatol Surg. 2013;39(12):1758–66.
3. DeLorenzi C. Complications of injectable fillers, part I. Aesthet Surg J. 2013;33(4):561–75.
4. Lee W, Yoon J-H, Koh I-S, Oh W, Kim K-W, Yang E-J. Clinical application of a new hyaluronic acid filler based on its rheological properties and the anatomical site of injection. Biomed Derm. 2018; 2(1):22.
5. Ozturk CN, Li Y, Tung R, Parker L, Piliang MP, Zins JE. Complications following injection of soft-tissue fillers. Aesthet Surg J. 2013;33(6):862–77.
6. Yang B, Guo X, Zang H, Liu J. Determination of modification degree in BDDE-modified hyaluronic acid hydrogel by SEC/MS. Carbohydr Polym. 2015;131:233–9.

Danger Zones of Filler Injections

4

Two distinct phenomena can occur when doctors inject filler for the first time. First, the doctor feels that the procedure is very easy and features an immediate response without any danger. Second, the doctor feels absolute fear about where to inject and how much filler to use. Both attitudes occur because of a lack of knowledge.

Filler injection is an easy but potentially dangerous procedure. However, it is not difficult to learn, so safety can be ensured with basic knowledge.

In this chapter, we will discuss facial danger zones and maximizing safety during filler injections.

4.1 Facial Danger Zones

Facial danger zones during filler injection are quite different from those during surgery. Surgery is basically a "destroying procedure," so danger zones include areas containing nerves and vessels. In comparison, fillers are basically used to fill an area, so inflated tissue properties are very important. Thus, we must consider the new concept of the facial danger zone in contrast to the surgical danger zone.

Location of danger zone during filler injection is shown in Table 4.1.

Table 4.1 Danger zones

Danger zones	
	Thick skin
	Subcutaneous layer
	Isolated area
	Foramen or notch of vessels

4.1.1 Thick Skin Area

Thick skin is hard and tough, so when the filler is injected, high resistance is encountered. Vessels between injected fillers and thick skin tend to increase the risk of necrosis compared to those in thin skin.

Studies have shown that the nasal tip, glabella, cheeks, and chin have relatively thick skins and that the most noticeable areas are the glabella and nasal tip (Table 4.2; Figs. 4.1, 4.2, 4.3, and 4.4). These two areas are most commonly treated with a filler, which tends to be injected superficially, and carry a higher risk of compression.

Table 4.2 Average skin thickness measurements

Site	Relative skin thickness index (±SD)
Upper lip	2.261 ± 0.539
Lower lip	2.259 ± 0.537
Philtrum	2.260 ± 0.375
Chin	3.144 ± 0.464
Upper eyelid	1 ± 0.000
Lower eyelid	2.189 ± 0.475
Forehead	2.850 ± 0.599
Right cheek	2.967 ± 0.661
Left cheek	3.226 ± 0.628
Malar eminence	2.783 ± 1.082
Submental	2.403 ± 0.500
Nasal tip	3.302 ± 0.491
Nasal dorsum	2.020 ± 0.478
Right neck	1.497 ± 0.824
Left neck	1.530 ± 0.764

Ha et al. [1]

© Springer Nature Singapore Pte Ltd. 2019
I. S. Koh, W. Lee, *Filler Complications*, https://doi.org/10.1007/978-981-13-6639-0_4

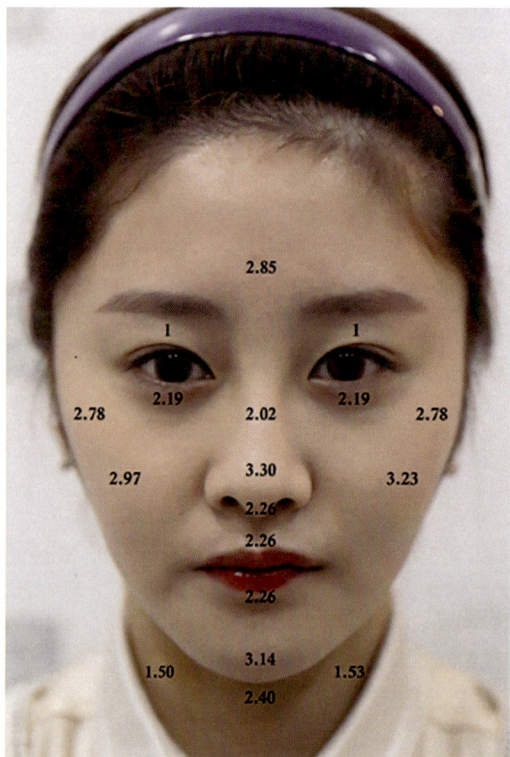

Fig. 4.1 Relative skin thicknesses of the face (upper eyelid = 1)

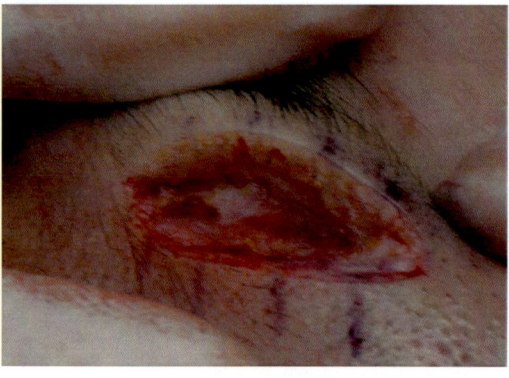

Fig. 4.2 Skin thickness of the glabella region. Glabella skin thickness during scar revision operation. The glabella region has thicker skin than the forehead area

4.1.2 Subcutaneous Layer

The arteries of the face run either from the internal carotid artery and run through the facial foramen or from the facial artery from the external carotid artery branches. They usually run near the bone or

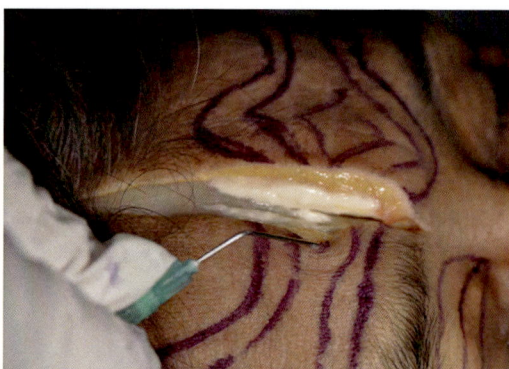

Fig. 4.3 Skin thicknesses of the forehead and glabella regions. Cadaveric dissection, perpendicular view. The glabella region has thicker skin than the forehead area

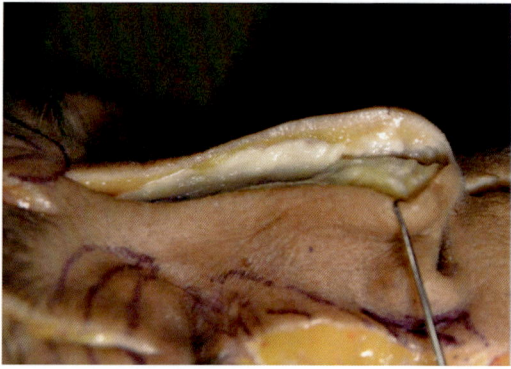

Fig. 4.4 Skin thickness of the nose. Cadaveric dissection. The nasal tip area has thicker skin than the nasal dorsum area. Clinicians must be aware of skin thickness during filler injections

through the foramen and run gradually to the superficial subcutaneous layers. There is a high risk of vessel injury when the filler is injected superficially because most vessels already run superficially.

The subcutaneous arteries have smaller diameters than the deep arteries, which increases the risk of ischemic necrosis when high-pressure filler is injected near the subcutaneous tissues. The risk is also increased when the filler is injected into thick skin.

Clinically important arteries include the:

- Supraorbital artery
- Supratrochlear artery
- Lateral nasal branch of the facial artery
- Dorsal nasal artery

4.1.2.1 The Supraorbital Artery

The supraorbital artery is a branch of the ophthalmic artery from the internal carotid artery that runs through the supraorbital notch or foramen and deeply under the frontalis muscles and/or runs superficially to create an anastomosis with the supratrochlear and superficial temporal arteries (Fig. 4.5).

The deep branch of the supraorbital artery might be located 12 mm above the orbital rim, so it should be approached very carefully. It can continue running deeply until 16–42 mm; therefore, the filler should be very carefully injected into the supraperiosteal layer. The skin is usually elevated at the squared area because of the corrugator muscle (Figs. 4.6 and 4.7).

4.1.2.2 The Supratrochlear Artery

The supratrochlear artery is a branch of the ophthalmic artery along with the supraorbital artery. The internal carotid artery branches from the ophthalmic and the supratrochlear artery posterior to the trochlear, perforates the medial orbital septum, and runs to the glabellar area. It tends to create an anastomosis with the contralateral supratrochlear artery.

After exiting the orbit, it runs superficially, so skin necrosis often occurs after injections are made to correct glabellar frown lines. This area is relatively thick, so it involves a higher risk of compression (Figs. 4.8, 4.9, 4.10, and 4.11).

4.1.2.3 The Lateral Nasal Artery

The lateral nasal artery is a branch of the facial artery at the level of the alar crease (Fig. 4.12). The facial artery tends to run deeper than the zygomaticus major and zygomaticus minor muscles and superficially to the levator labii superioris and levator labii superioris alaeque nasi muscles. Thus, the lateral nasal artery is located in the subcutaneous layer (Fig. 4.13).

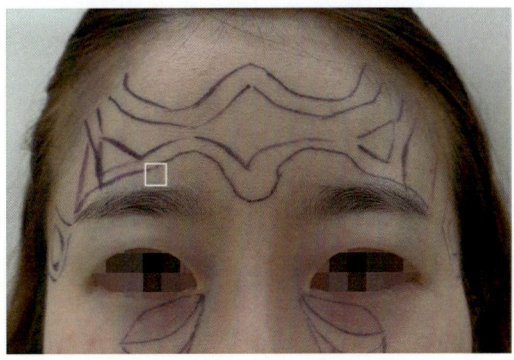

Fig. 4.6 Location of supraorbital artery perforation. Supraorbital artery perforation location (squared)

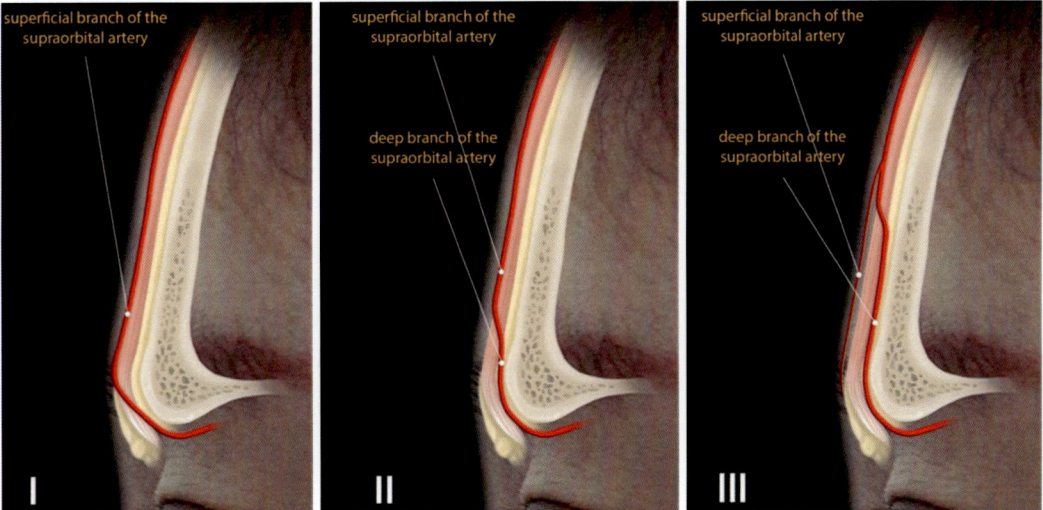

Fig. 4.5 Classification of the supraorbital artery. The supraorbital artery tends to run subcutaneously in types I and II but tends to run deep to the postfrontalis muscle in type III

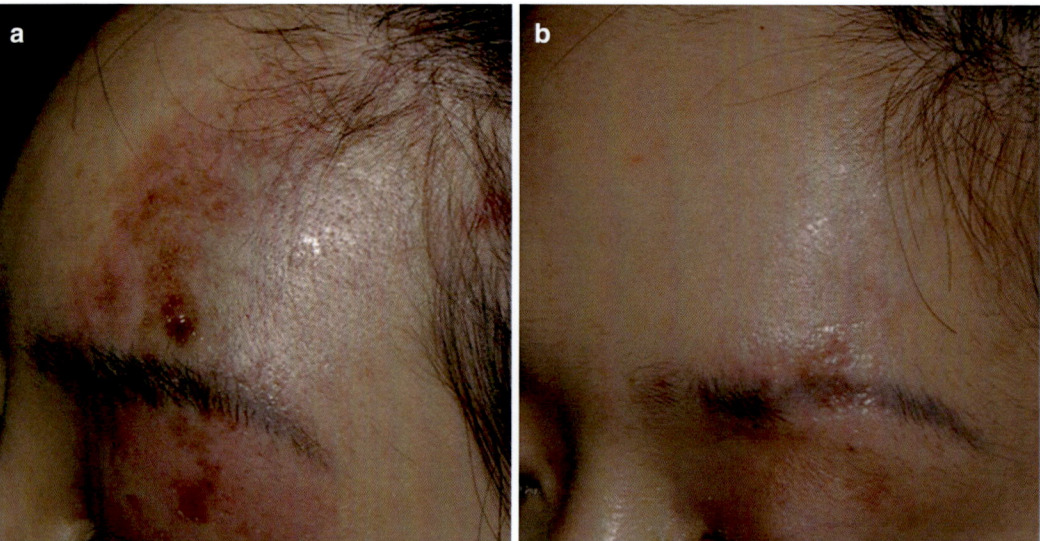

Fig. 4.7 Damaged supraorbital artery. (**a**) Three days post-calcium hydroxyapatite filler injection into the forehead. The territory of the supraorbital artery has been damaged. Damaged areas might have sequelae. (**b**) Two weeks after treatment

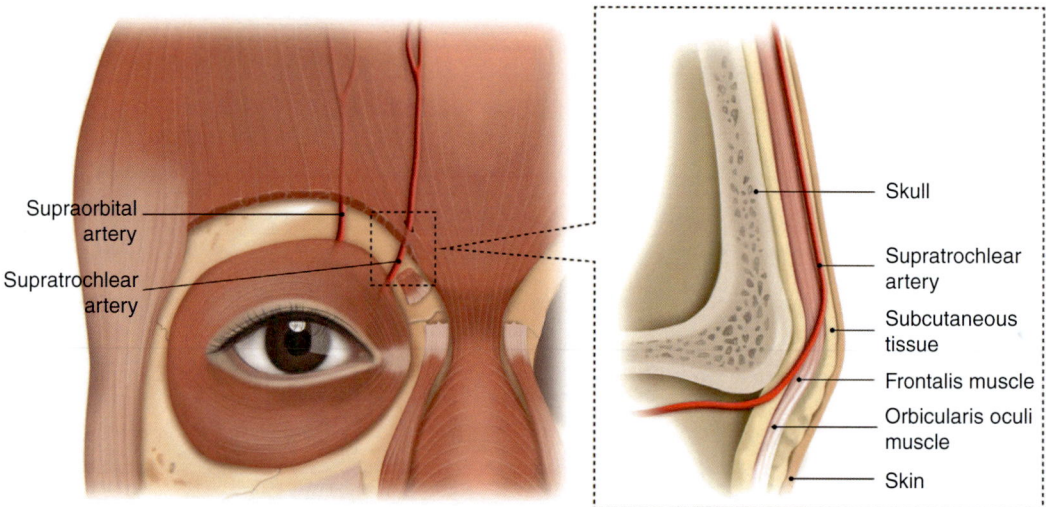

Fig. 4.8 Location of the supratrochlear artery. The superficial branch of the supratrochlear artery runs through the subcutaneous plane (dotted square); therefore, subcutaneous injections into the glabellar frown line should be given carefully. The superficial branch is dominant

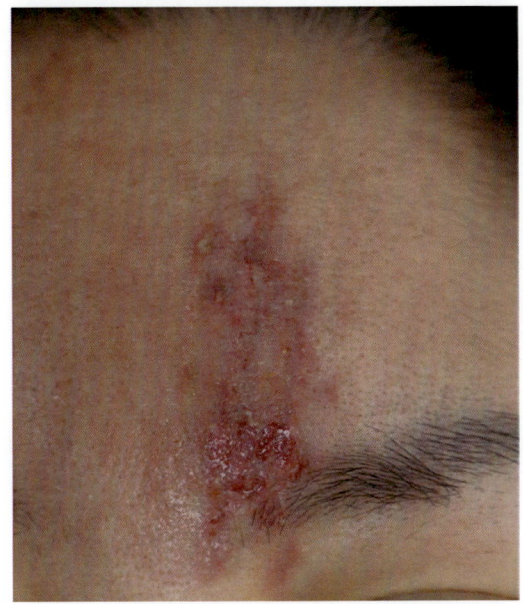

Fig. 4.9 Supratrochlear artery damage. Five days after filler injection. Skin damages along with supratrochlear artery territory. This area is relatively thick skin

The lateral nasal artery is susceptible to injury during filler injection for nasolabial fold correction because it tends to run superficial to the subcutaneous layer between the nasolabial fold and the upper part of the nasolabial fold, called the premaxillary or infraorbital region. When injections are made into the subcutaneous layer in this area, there is a high possibility of damaging this artery (Fig. 4.14).

When the facial artery is constricted due to an infraorbital nerve block by epinephrine anesthesia, the superior labial, lateral nasal, and dorsal nasal arteries could be constricted simultaneously (Fig. 4.15). Therefore, it is likely to affect the adjacent vessels because they create an anastomosis.

The author's preinjection design is shown in Fig. 4.16. The lateral nasal artery runs subcutaneously (arrow) and is commonly damaged. Most doctors do not augment their work right away, but over time, they try to perfect their results by

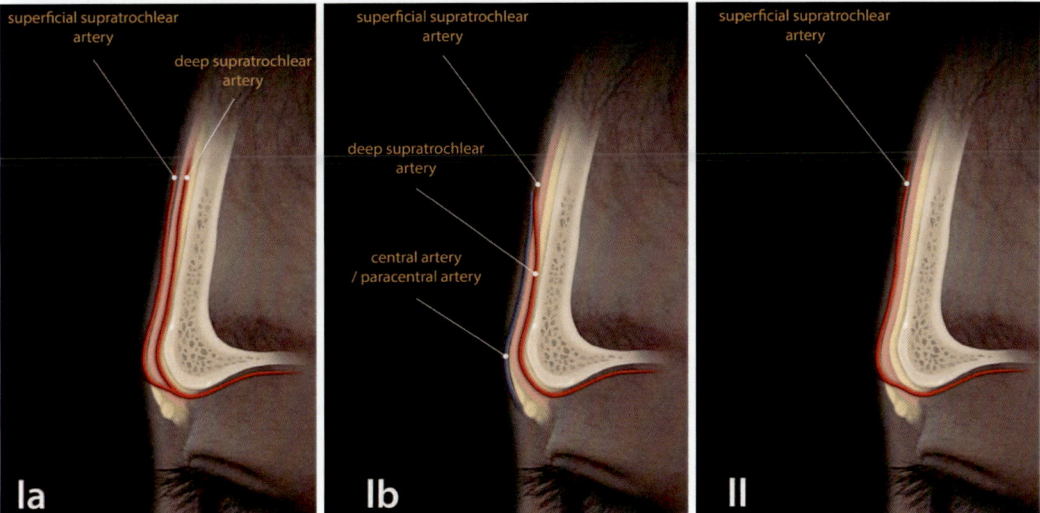

Fig. 4.10 Supratrochlear artery pathway. There is no deep branch of the supratrochlear artery like type II, but 55% exist deep branch (type Ia + Ib). Type Ib shows superficial branch anastomosis with central artery. To inject into the supraperiosteal layer is not a completely safe method because the supratrochlear artery and supraorbital artery might have deep branches

Fig. 4.11 Location of supratrochlear artery; cadaveric view. Deep branches of the supratrochlear artery are seen. Filler injection into this artery can cause serious problems

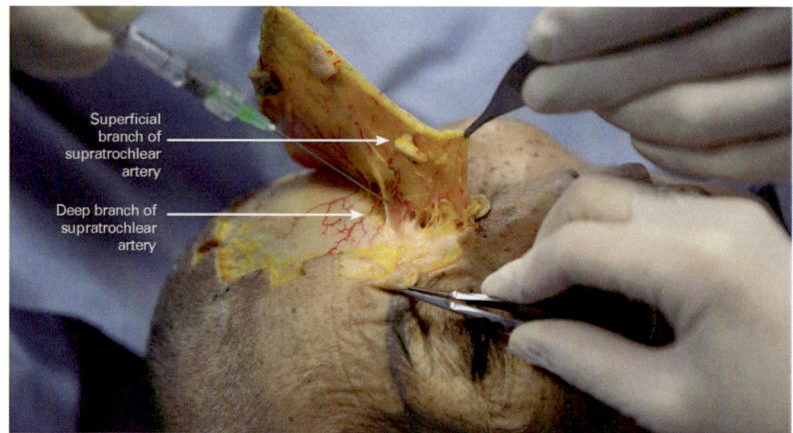

Fig. 4.12 The lateral nasal artery and adjacent arteries. The facial artery branches into the lateral nasal artery at the level of the alar crease, followed by the angular nasal artery, and creates an anastomosis with the dorsal nasal artery

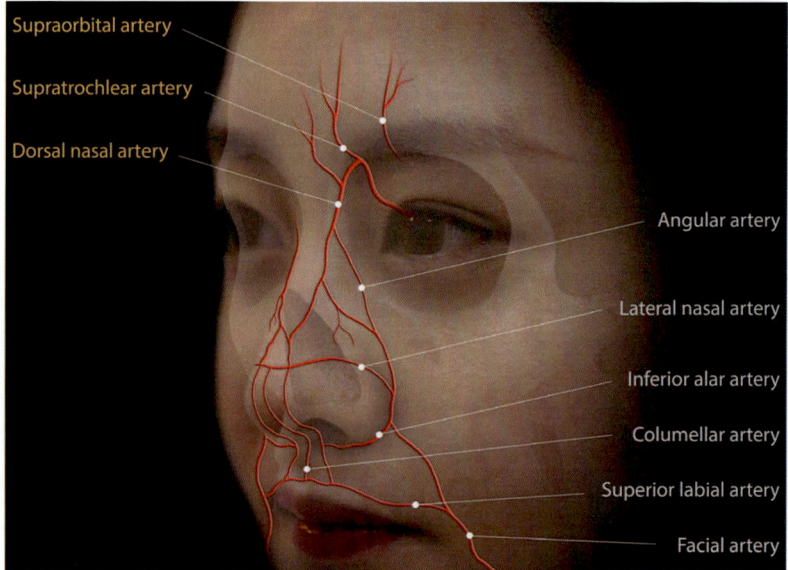

injecting into this area and compromise the vessels (Figs. 4.17, 4.18, 4.19, 4.20, and 4.21).

4.1.2.4 The Dorsal Nasal Artery

The dorsal nasal artery is the ophthalmic artery branch from the internal carotid artery. It supplies the nose after perforating above the medial palpebral ligament at the orbit and then creates an anastomosis with the contralateral dorsal nasal

artery and the lateral nasal artery. The relationship between these arteries is shown in Fig. 4.22. This vessel also runs through the subcutaneous layer; thus, a superficial injection may cause vascular compromise (Fig. 4.22).

Four arteries have been described. The supraorbital, supratrochlear, and dorsal nasal arteries arise from the internal carotid artery, while the lateral nasal artery arises from the external

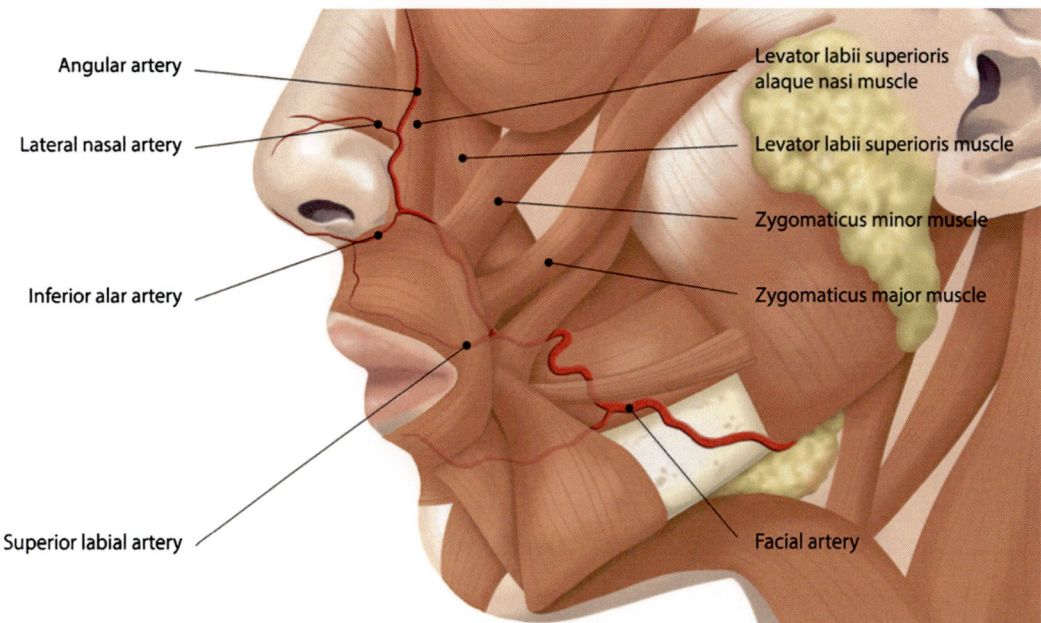

Angular artery

Lateral nasal artery

Inferior alar artery

Superior labial artery

Levator labii superioris
alaque nasi muscle

Levator labii superioris muscle

Zygomaticus minor muscle

Zygomaticus major muscle

Facial artery

Fig. 4.13 Location of the lateral nasal artery. The facial artery runs deep to the zygomaticus major and minor muscles and runs superficially to the subcutaneous layer at the level of the levator labii superioris and levator labii superioris alaeque nasi muscles. The lateral nasal artery is branched

Fig. 4.14 The lateral nasal artery: cadaver view. The lateral nasal artery is located within the subcutaneous layer (arrow); therefore, it is susceptible to injury during subcutaneous filler injection

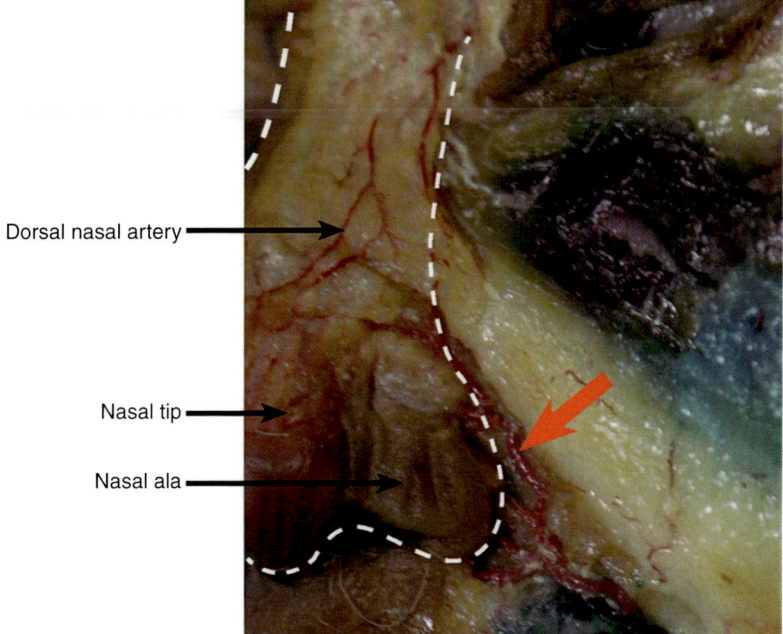

Dorsal nasal artery

Nasal tip

Nasal ala

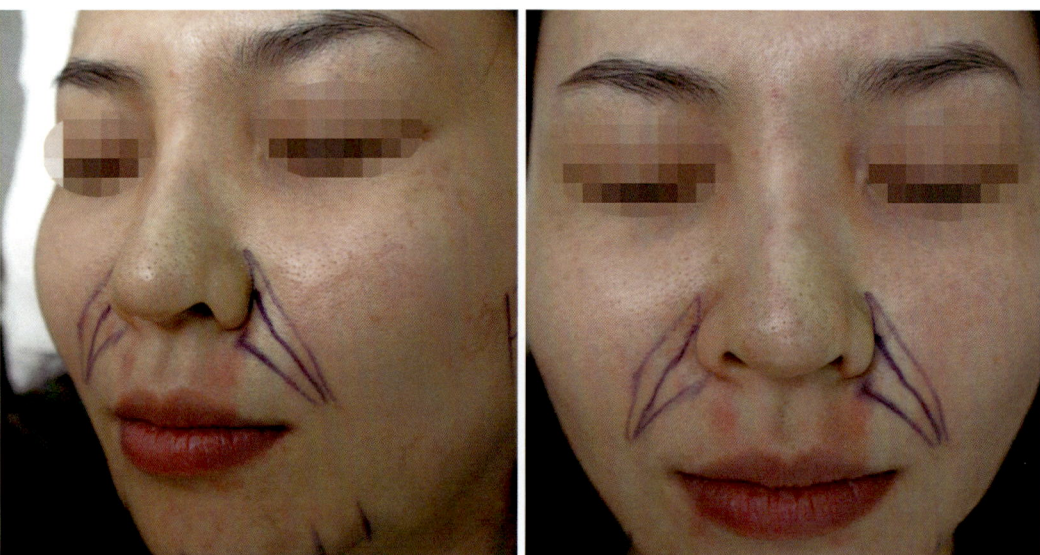

Fig. 4.15 Blanching phenomenon after infraorbital nerve block. The lateral nasal artery and superior labial artery territories are blanched due to the infraorbital nerve block of epinephrine anesthesia

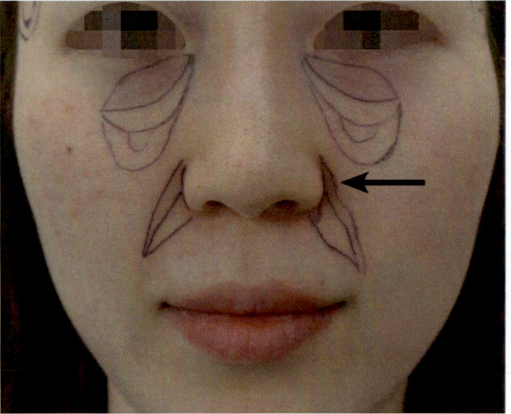

Fig. 4.16 Author's preinjection design for correcting the nasolabial fold. Most common compromised place because the lateral nasal artery runs subcutaneously (arrow pointed)

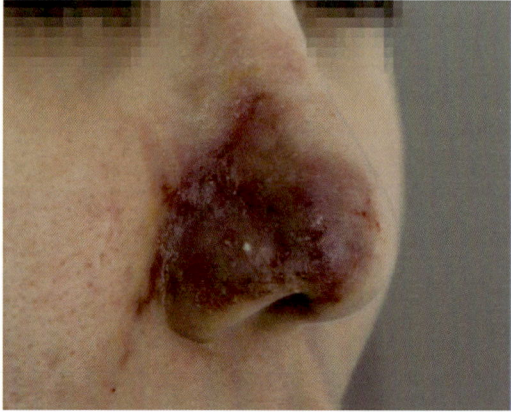

Fig. 4.17 Vascular compromise after filler injection into the nasolabial fold. Classical vascular embolism of the lateral nasal artery 4 days after the injection of hyaluronic acid filler to correct the nasolabial fold

carotid artery. The three vessels arising from the internal carotid artery are important because their compromise could cause the most tragic filler complication, blindness induced by retrograde filler injection (Fig. 4.23).

The lateral nasal and angular arteries also create an anastomosis with the dorsal nasal artery, so any filler injections made near the internal carotid artery should be done very carefully. These arteries tend to run through the subcutaneous layer, so avoid making injections into the superficial layer or use a large-diameter needle such as a 23G to prevent a high-pressure injection. If a high-pressure filler injection is made and filler is

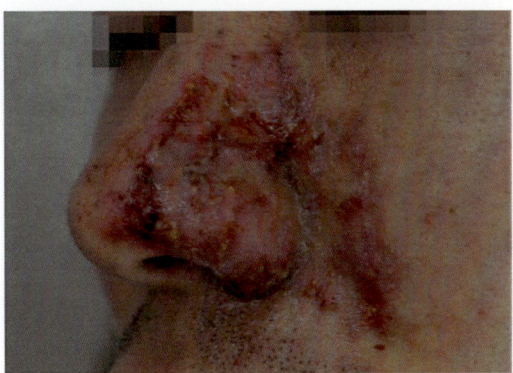

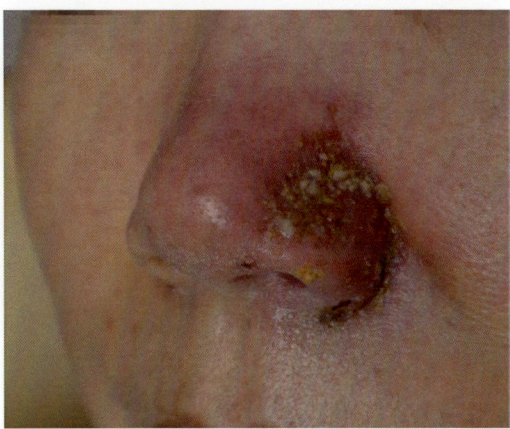

Fig. 4.18 Vascular compromise after filler injection into the nasolabial fold. One week after the injection of the hyaluronic acid filler into the nasolabial fold. Wound discharge, pustules, and eschar formation are visible after vascular compromise without treatment. Extensive wound damage is visible at the lateral nasal and angular artery territories

Fig. 4.20 Vascular compromise after the injection of filler into the nasolabial fold. Three days after injection of the hyaluronic acid filler into the nasolabial fold. Multiple pustules at the alar crease and surrounding inflammation are visible due to lateral nasal artery compromise

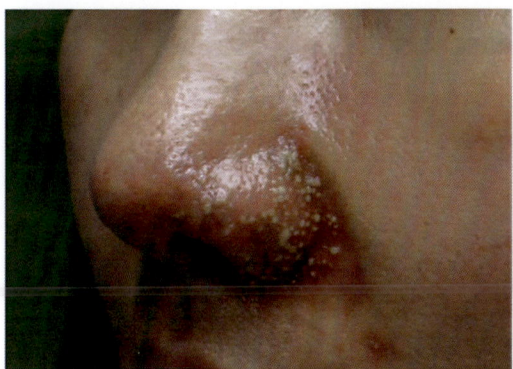

Fig. 4.19 Vascular compromise after injection of filler into the nasolabial fold. Three days after the injection of hyaluronic acid filler into the nasolabial fold. Multiple pustules are visible in the territory of the lateral nasal artery

injected retrogradely, serious complications such as blindness may occur (Fig. 4.24).

4.1.3   Isolated Area

Some regions have different skin properties and anatomical structures. One example of such a region is the nasal tip, which is composed of thicker skin than the nasal dorsum and has a

unique structure in which the subcutaneous tissue is tightly bonded with the SMAS layers. This area is important because pressure that is introduced with injections cannot be diffused, which increases the risk of necrosis (Fig. 4.25).

In contrast, the dorsum area is at relatively low risk because its skin is thinner and loosely connected between subcutaneous tissues and the SMAS. When making injections into the nasal tip area, it is very important to inject 70% of the maximum amount to decrease the pressure. Especially when injecting fillers that tend to cause swelling, such as calcium hydroxyapatite filler and polycaprolactone filler, it is important to consider injecting only 60% of the maximum amount.

Regarding these properties, when injecting filler into the nasal tip area, clinicians should follow up with the patient the next day to check for pain, color changes, and swelling; if problems are noted, early decompression is very important.

4.1.4   Foramen

A foramen is a hole through which vessels perforate the bone. Important vessels include the

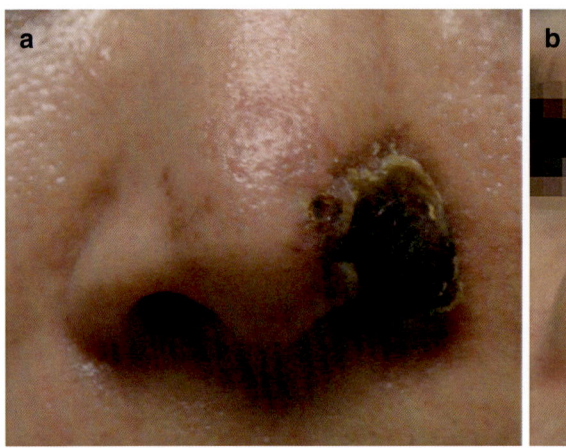
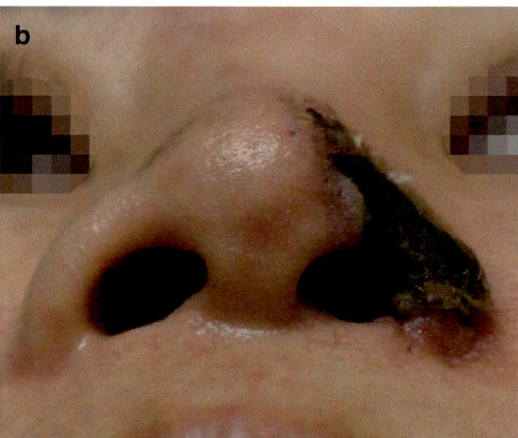

Fig. 4.21 Full-thickness skin necrosis induced by vascular compromise after the injection of filler into the nasolabial fold. One month after the injection of hyaluronic acid filler into the nasolabial fold. Full-thickness skin necrosis occurred in the left nasal alar area due to the lack of appropriate treatment after lateral nasal artery compromise. (**a**) Frontal view. (**b**) Worm's eye view

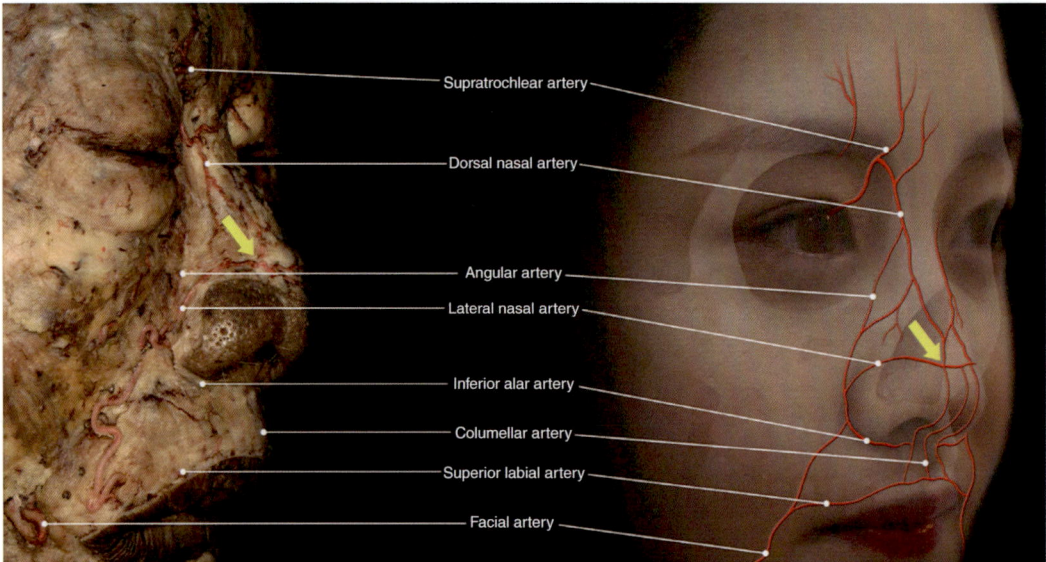

Fig. 4.22 The dorsal nasal artery and adjacent arteries. The dorsal nasal artery creates an anastomosis with the lateral nasal artery (arrow) and runs through the subcutaneous layer. The nasal vessels are located in the subcutaneous layer, which is superficial to the superficial muscular aponeurotic system (SMAS) layer

Fig. 4.23 The external carotid artery versus the internal carotid artery. The external carotid artery branches are drawn in black, while the internal carotid artery branches, the ophthalmic artery, and related branched arteries are drawn in red. The supraorbital, supratrochlear, dorsal nasal arteries arise from the internal carotid artery and are important

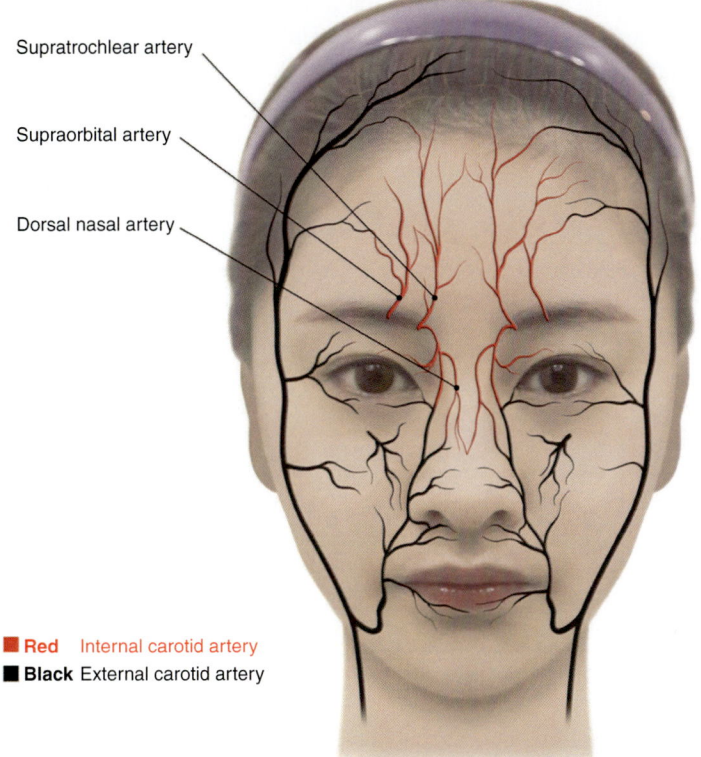

Supratrochlear artery

Supraorbital artery

Dorsal nasal artery

■ **Red**   Internal carotid artery
■ **Black** External carotid artery

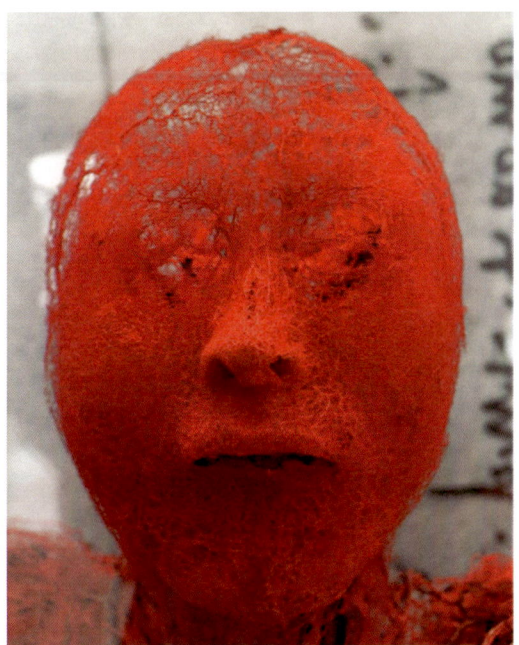

Fig. 4.24 Facial vascular model created by injecting latex into a cadaver. It is very difficult to avoid vessels during injections because so many vessels are located very closely together, particularly in the subcutaneous layer, so it is important to make injections into relatively avascular planes. (Photographed at China)

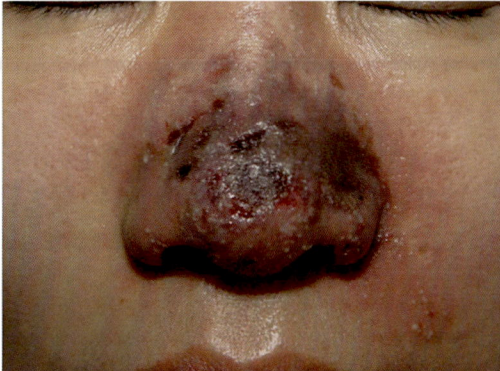

Fig. 4.25 Skin necrosis in the nasal tip. Skin necrosis first visible 3 days after calcium hydroxyapatite filler injection into the nasal tip, where it tends to progress quickly

supraorbital artery from the supraorbital foramen and the infraorbital artery from the infraorbital foramen.

The regions in which vessels perforate should be approached very carefully because vessels can be damaged if injections are made nearby. The danger is increased because the foramen holds the vessel, similar to holding a vessel in one's hand. This area is also important when a local anesthesia is injected because nerves can be damaged as well.

4.2   Safe Zones

Safe zones are opposites of danger zones (Table 4.3). Smooth and thin skins can disperse pressure by allowing skin surfaces to expand.

Just above periosteal or perichondrial layer is an avascular plane, a target layer for surgery. For the same reason, it is safe for filler injection.

The nasal tip is an isolated high-risk region; in contrast, the nasal dorsum area can disperse pressure when filler is injected, making it relatively safe. When one pinches and moves the nasal tip skin and the nasal dorsum skin, the differences become clear as the nasal tip feels like a lump and the nasal dorsum glides smoothly. This phenomenon occurs because of differences in the tight bonding between the subcutaneous tissue and the SMAS.

Locations where multiple vessels create an anastomosis could be safe places because of collateral circulation. These places are the lips and eyelids, which are at relatively lower risk of vascular compromise.

Table 4.3 Safe filler injection zones

Safe zones	Thin, soft skin
	Supraperiosteal layer
	Non-isolated area
	Multiple anastomosis vascular network
Relative safe region	Muscular layer
	Lesser anastomosis vascular network

The muscular layer is also known to be relatively safe because it can disperse the pressure, but it has many vessels, so it is not completely safe.

4.3   Danger Zone Characteristics and Injection Techniques

Danger zones are shown in Fig. 4.26.

4.3.1   Glabella

The glabella region contains thick skin, and the supratrochlear artery (arising from the internal carotid artery) is located within the subcutaneous layer. Therefore, localized skin necrosis due to thick skin or blindness and cerebral infarction due to embolism can occur.

To prevent these complications, minimal amounts of filler should be injected into a supratrochlear artery location if possible. Glabellar

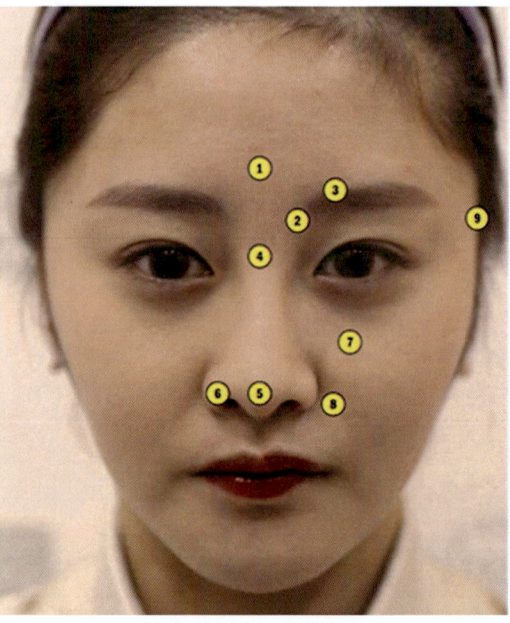

Fig. 4.26 Danger zones for filler injection. 1 Glabella, 2 Supratrochlear artery perforating orbital septum, 3 Supraorbital artery perforating supraorbital foramen or notch, 4 Nasal root, 5 Nasal tip, 6 Nose alar, 7 Infraorbital foramen, 8 Nasolabial fold, 9 Temple

wrinkles tend to be in the same location as the supratrochlear vessels, so care should be taken.

Some glabellar wrinkles are located in the proximal regions where the supratrochlear artery perforates the orbital septum, so special care is required for corrections made in this region (Fig. 4.27).

The authors like to use Koh's block masonry technique to correct glabellar wrinkles (Fig. 4.28).

When injecting into this area, the needle should be advanced and aspirated, and the injection should be made gently with minimal pressure using a large-diameter needle such as a 23G. The first injection should be made into the preperiosteal layer to create the foundation for the whole procedure, while the last injection should be made into the subcutaneous layer. Injections made into the subcutaneous layer require more attention. When injecting into the subcutaneous layer, clinicians must advance and aspirate the needle to check for blood and then make the injection carefully to ensure low skin tension.

Hyaluronic acid fillers tend to cause water retention and expand, so 70% of the maximum amount should be injected.

4.3.2 The Forehead

The supraorbital artery also arises from the internal carotid artery, so filler injected into the vessel could cause blindness or cerebral infarction (Figs. 4.5 and 4.6).

The supraorbital artery has a superficial branch and a deep branch (Fig. 4.5). It runs at subcutaneous layer, and it is safer to inject filler at the supraperiosteal layer. However, even in supraperiosteal injection, it is not completely safe because as in type III deep branch, it could run into the supraperiosteal layer until 16–42 mm from the supraorbital rim and until 12 mm at supraperiosteal layer. Therefore, injections should not be given below 12 mm and should be done carefully for 12–42 mm.

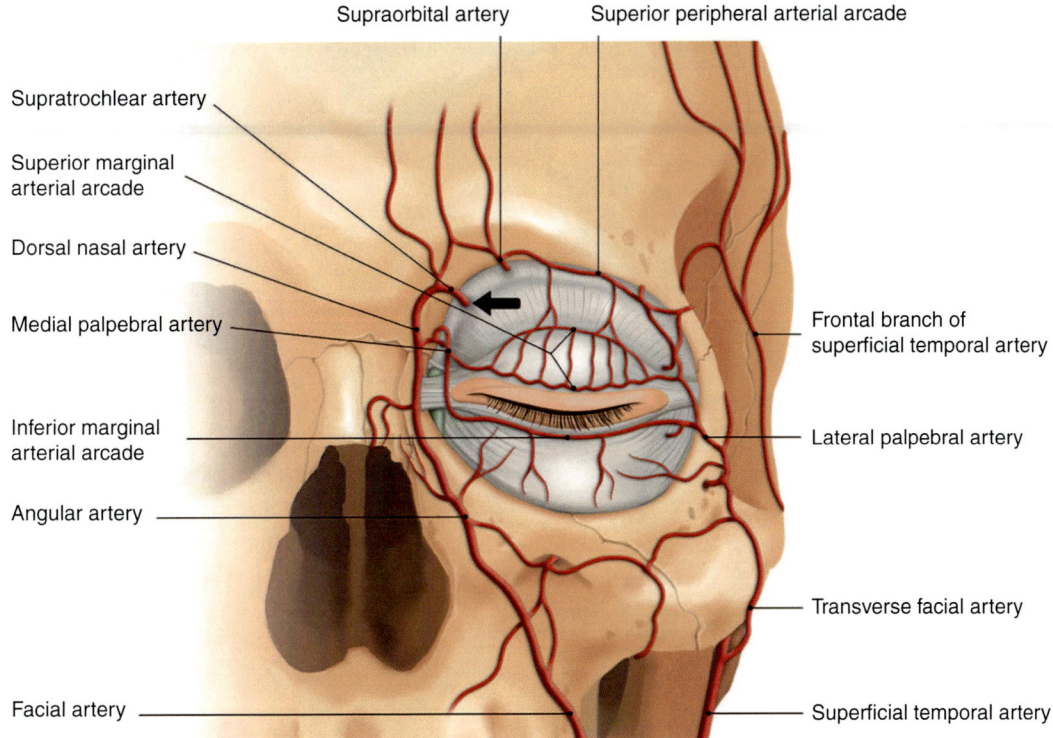

Fig. 4.27 The supratrochlear artery perforating the orbital septum. Supratrochlear artery perforating the orbital septum (arrow)

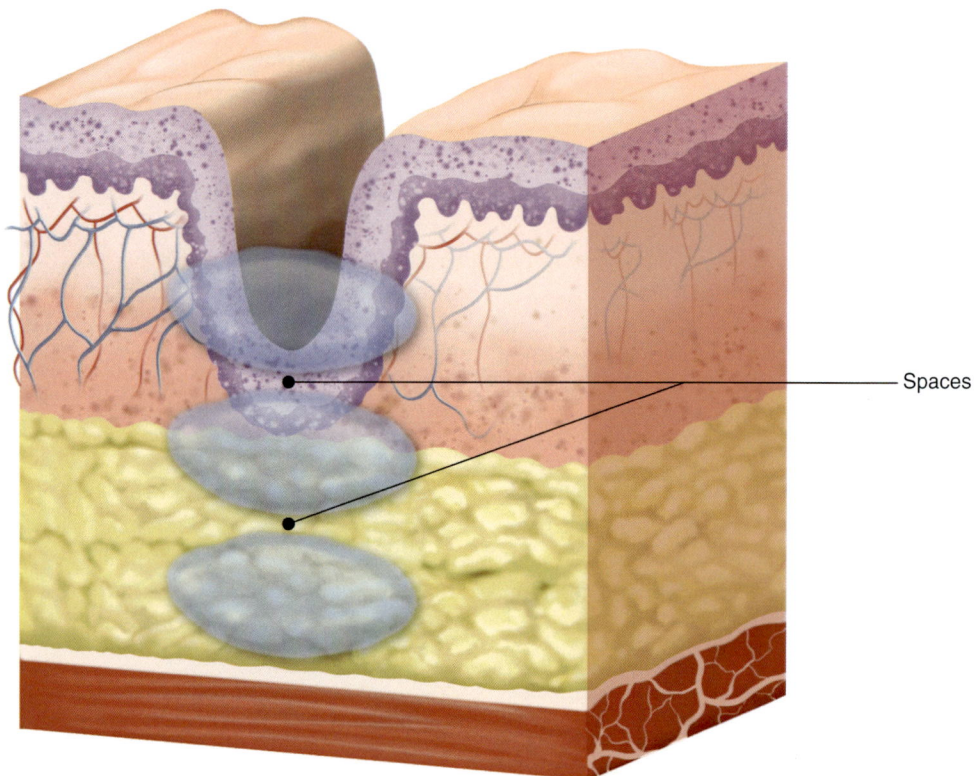

Spaces

Fig. 4.28 Koh's block masonry technique. Filler injection layer by layer as in the block masonry technique to effectively correct wrinkles using a small amount of filler

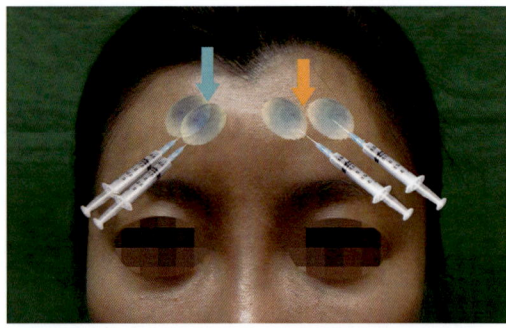

Fig. 4.29 Koh's expanding technique. A useful technique for wide area augmentation, such as the forehead or temple. First, inject the filler to make one space, and then inject the overlapping spaces to ensure continuous and smooth contour line (blue arrow). It is difficult to make continuous smooth contour by injection into the solitary space (orange arrow)

We will introduce Koh's expanding technique that minimizes vessel injuries and allows even injection to a wide area such as the forehead (Fig. 4.29).

Koh's expanding technique is useful to augment wide areas such as the forehead or temple. One space is first made with a long needle, and overlapping space is injected to make continuous and smooth contour. When injecting the overlapping area, injection should be first made in the margin. Then the first injected area is compressed with the other hand when injecting the next one, to expand filler to the opposite direction.

Its principle is based on hydrodissection technique, which involves dissection by water pressure. The needle does not need to locate where to augment, but filler is forwarding first; therefore, it can reduce chances of vessel damage.

Injection by a preexisting method is difficult for augmentation of a wide area such as the forehead. Using a small needle, new injection should be made solitary from the first injection, resulting in two solitary augmented regions. It is very difficult to inject between them. Moreover, there is an increase of vessel damage when injection is done many times.

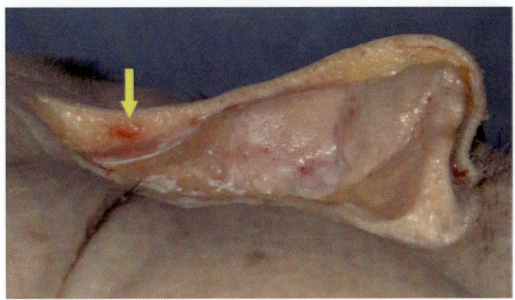

Fig. 4.30 Cross section of the nose. Vessels are visible in the subcutaneous layer, which is superficial to the SMAS at the nasal root region (yellow arrow). Filler can be injected into the dorsal nasal artery in the subcutaneous layer

4.3.3   The Nasal Root

The nasal root region is supplied by the dorsal nasal artery, and this artery arises from the internal carotid artery, which leads to the risk of blindness and cerebral infarction.

Recently, there have been cases of blindness during nasal augmentation by filler injections because of embolism of dorsal nasal artery and regurgitation to ophthalmic artery. One of the common procedures for filler injection in Asian is nasal augmentation, and it is very important to concern about embolism.

Nasal root area is not an isolated region compared to the nasal tip, and the skin is thinner than the skin of nasal tip. Also, the skin is not tightly connected with the SMAS layer. Therefore, the nasal root is a relatively safer region for skin necrosis by compression. However, there is a higher tendency of injection to the subcutaneous region to make sharper shape nose, and this phenomena could increase the risk of embolism. Moreover, by using along cannula, this risk has been increased (Figs. 4.22 and 4.30).

To prevent this complication, it is important to use a large-diameter cannula or needle (e.g., 23G), making it easier to deliver the needle tip to the desired layer. However, many injectors like to use cannula. A cannula has a blunt tip and is easy to localize within the subcutaneous layer, which

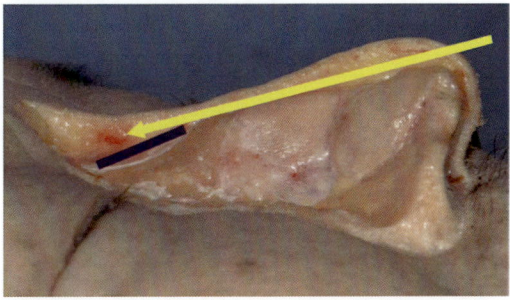

Fig. 4.31 Nasal augmentation cannula injection pathway. Nasal bone location and angle are highlighted by the blue line. When using a long cannula from the infralobule approach, the cannula tip enters the subcutaneous layer at the nasal root area (yellow arrow). When a dorsal nasal artery embolism occurs, it can cause blindness or cerebral infarction. Thus, at the junction of the nasal bone and the septal cartilage, it is important to control the cannula tip deeply within the supraperiosteal layer

features less resistance. Thus, when a cannula is used, it is important to control the cannula tip. A cannula larger than 21G should be used to more easily control its direction. When the cannula tip has reached the nasal bone and septal cartilage junction, the cannula tip was located in the supraperiosteal layer, meaning that the needle can scratch the bone prior to the injection (Fig. 4.31).

4.3.4 Nasal Tip

The nasal tip typically contains thick skin that is tightly attached to the SMAS. It is a solitary region, so when a large amount of filler is injected into it, the pressure cannot be dispersed and skin necrosis may occur. In particular, the subcutaneous layer is not soft, so it is vulnerable to skin necrosis.

The injector may tend to augment the sharp nasal tip and tend to inject filler into the subcutaneous layer, where the lateral nasal artery is susceptible to injury. Considering maximal tension as 100%, an amount lower than 70% should be injected. The other 30% should remain to account for injection swelling and water retention. Injections between the two alar cartilages are safe (Fig. 4.32).

When injecting into the nasal tip, it is important not to create a wide tip. The authors like to use a 23G needle when augmenting only the nasal tip.

4.3.5 Ala Nasi (Wing of the Nose)

The ala nasi is the place more rigid than the nasal tip area, so filler injections into this region might cause localized necrosis. The skin is so rigid that even temporarily corrected grooves might be visible again within 2 weeks after treatment.

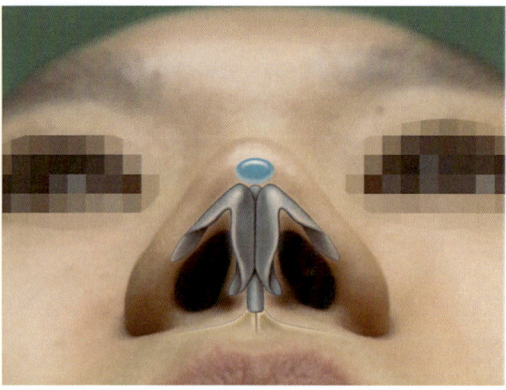

Fig. 4.32 Filler injection location at the nasal tip. Filler should be injected near the two areas of alar cartilage to prevent spreading to the skin

4.3.6 Infraorbital Foramen

The use of filler for premaxillary augmentation is increasing nowadays. The anatomy near the infraorbital foramen is shown in Fig. 4.33. It is usually safe to inject filler into the suborbicularis oculi fat (SOOF) layer (Fig. 4.34).

When injecting filler into the deepest part, one should avoid the infraorbital foramen, where the infraorbital nerve and vessel perforate. This is likely to hold vessels and nerves down one side, so puncture here is highly dangerous. The infraorbital foramen is directed downward and one step from the infraorbital rim, so it is safer to make the injection in the downward direction rather than the upward direction (Figs. 4.35 and 4.36).

4.3.7 Nasolabial Fold

The nasolabial fold is one of the most common filler injection places. Since many procedures are performed, many complications also occur. The most noticeable vessel is the lateral nasal artery, which runs from the facial artery branch at the alar crease.

The facial artery tends to run deep to the zygomaticus major and minor muscles and run superficially to the levator labii superioris and levator labii superioris alaeque nasi muscles. The lateral nasal artery is located in the subcutaneous layer. Of course, not every human has the same arterial system, but the subcutaneous layer should be considered.

This vessel tends to be damaged during nasolabial fold correction. The lateral nasal artery crosses from the premaxillary or infraorbital region to the upper part of the nasolabial fold. Thus, injections into this region tend to damage the vessel (Figs. 4.13 and 4.14). The most common location is indicated by an arrow in Fig. 4.37.

The lateral nasal artery tends to be injured in the area indicated by the arrow. Alar rim necrosis or nasal tip necrosis could occur, while blindness or cerebral infarction might occur due to dorsal nasal artery embolisms that connect with the angular artery. Such damage leads to alar rim

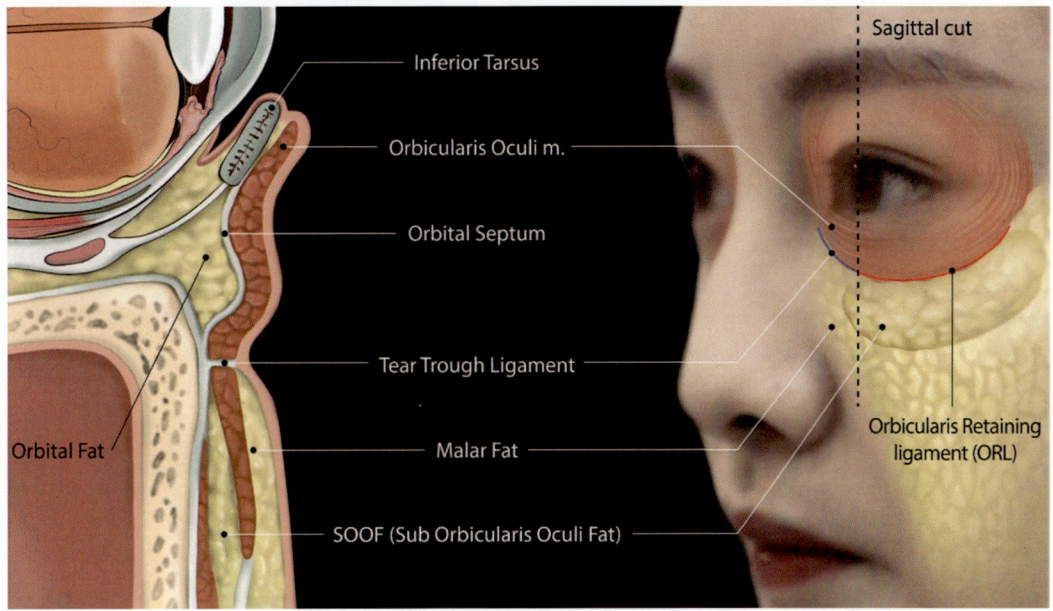

Fig. 4.33 Anatomy near the infraorbital foramen. Premaxillary area augmentation usually targets the SOOF layer

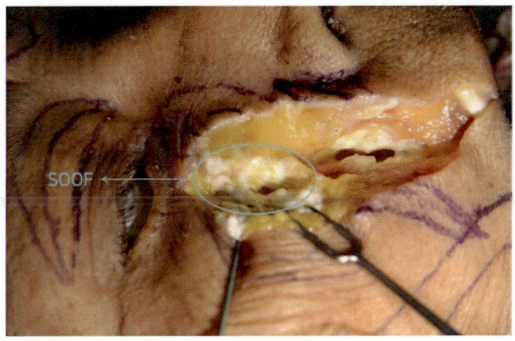

Fig. 4.34 Cadaveric dissection of the premaxillary region. White filler is visible in the SOOF layer

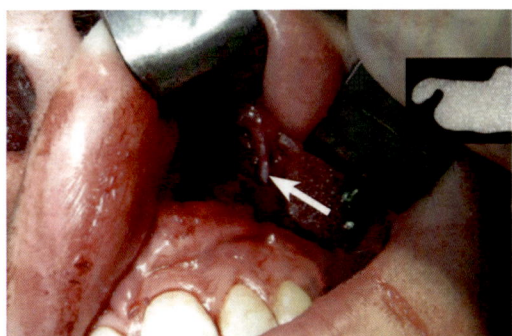

Fig. 4.35 Infraorbital artery perforating the infraorbital foramen. Intraoral view of the infraorbital artery (arrow), which is likely to be injured if injections are made directly into the infraorbital foramen

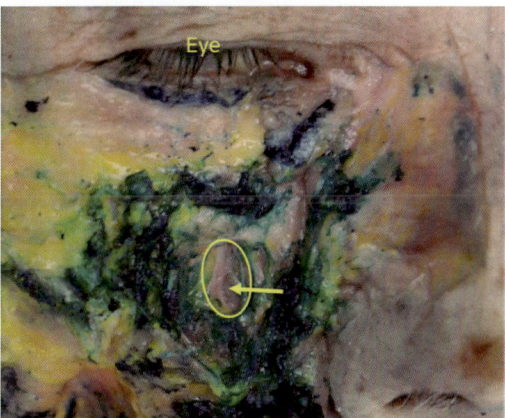

Fig. 4.36 Cadaveric view of the infraorbital nerve and vessel. Infraorbital nerve and vessels are indicated by the arrow after SOOF removal. The blue color dye indicates where filler was injected for the premaxillary augmentation

necrosis or nasal tip necrosis, while blindness or cerebral infarction might occur due to dorsal nasal artery embolism (Fig. 4.12).

Lateral nasal injuries tend to be made by experienced rather than beginner injectors since doctors with sufficient experience and confidence making filler injections tend to achieve better results and make injections into the subcutaneous layer where the lateral nasal artery is located.

Thus, when correcting a nasolabial fold, always remember the pathway of the lateral nasal artery.

4.3.8   Temple

The temple's anatomy is quite complicated. We define the temple area from the superior temporal septum to the zygomatic arch, and it contains many different layers. From the outside, there is the skin, subcutaneous layer, superficial temporal fascia (temporoparietal fascia), innominate fascia

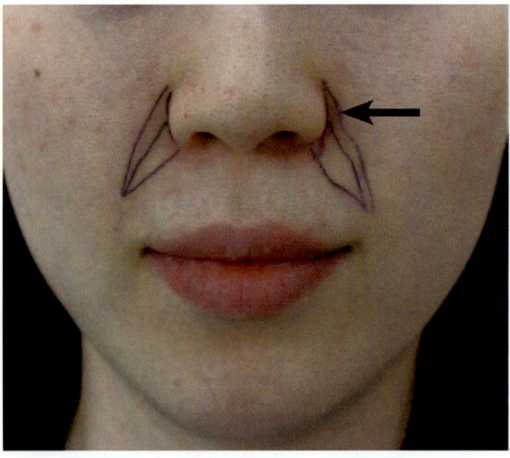

Fig. 4.37 Danger zone of nasolabial fold injection

and parotid temporal fascia, deep temporal fascia superficial layer, deep temporal fascia deep layer, temporalis muscle, and temporal bone. The layer should be compared with other facial regions (Table 4.4).

Theoretically, we can inject soft-tissue filler into four spaces: (1) subcutaneous layer; (2) space between the superficial temporal fascia and the deep temporal fascia; (3) space between the superficial layer and the deep layer of the deep temporal fascia; and (4) under the temporalis muscle (Fig. 4.38).

The first space is the subcutaneous layer, which is a superficial fat compartment that consists of the lateral temporal cheek compartment and the lateral orbital compartment. The superficial temporal vein and the sentinel vein are located in this layer. Veins can be detected in thin skin, but when torn, severe bruising might occur. When injected deeply, the superficial temporal artery or zygomatico-orbital artery can also be damaged. We recently used near-infrared technology to detect veins and avoid injuring them (Fig. 4.39).

The second space is that between the superficial temporal fascia and the deep temporal fascia. This area can be divided by the inferior temporal septum into the upper temporal compartment and the lower temporal compartment. The upper temporal compartment is a relatively safe region, and the lower temporal compartment should be con-

Table 4.4 Facial layers

Layer	Scalp	Forehead	Temple		Cheek(lateral)	Cheek(anterior)
1	Skin	Skin	Skin		Skin	Skin
2	Connective tissue	Superficial fat layer	Superficial fat layer lateral temporal cheek compartment		Superficial fat layer	Superficial fat layer
3	Aponeurotica	*Frontalis muscle*	*Superficial temporal fascia*		*SMAS Platysma*	Mimetic muscle
4	Loose areolar tissue	Subgaleal space ROOF Galeal fat pad	Loose areolar tissue		Sub-SMAS plane Premasseteric space	Deep fat layer Prezygomatic and premaxillary space SOOF
			Innominate fascia	Parotid temporal fascia		
5	Periosteum	Periosteum	Deep temporal fascia Temporal fat pad		Parotid masseteric fascia	
6			Temporalis muscle		Parotid gland Masseter muscle Buccal fat	

SMAS superficial muscular aponeurotic system

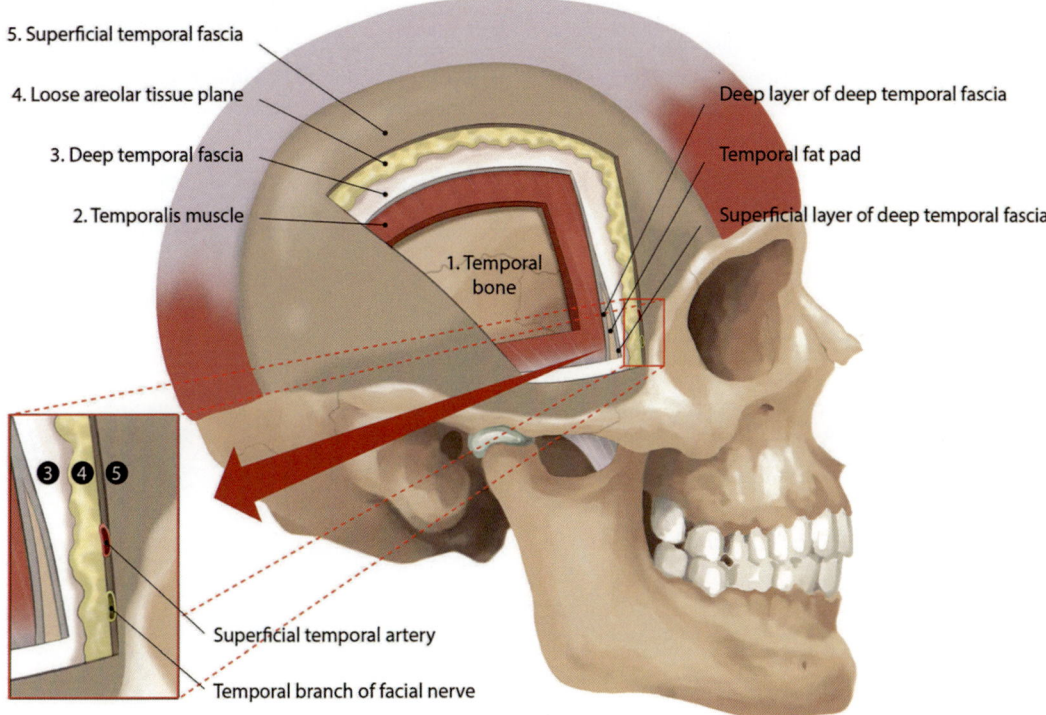

Fig. 4.38 Temple layers

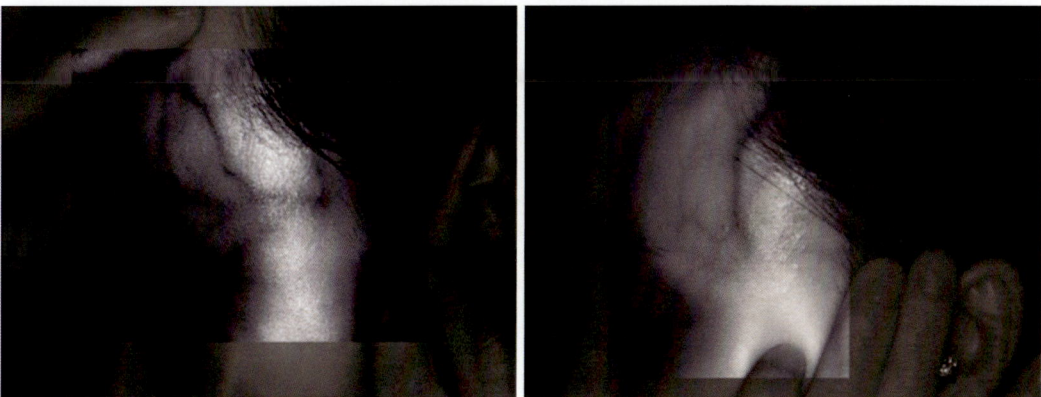

Fig. 4.39 High-resolution near-infrared illumination of the sentinel vein and superficial temporal vein. Anatomic variation between patients is demonstrated [2]

sidered the deep temporal vein perforating branch. To use a cannula, we must puncture the superficial temporal fascia and inject filler into this area. The deep temporal fascia is very hard, making it difficult to perforate by a cannula; in contrast, it is quite easy to inject into the upper temporal compartment.

The third space is that between the superficial layer and deep layer of the deep temporal fascia, which includes the temporal fat pad. The problem is that we cannot approach this area using a cannula because we must perforate the deep temporal fascia superficial layer, which is difficult to do with a cannula. When using a needle, we cannot estimate this layer. Also, if we inject a little deeper than the deep temporal fascia, we may encounter the muscle and buccal fat pad temporal extension, at which point the filler might migrate to the buccal portion.

The fourth space is that under the temporalis muscle. It is a relatively avascular space, but it might involve multiple problems: (1) Temporalis muscle is a mastication muscle that is firmly attached to the temporal bone, so filler should be injected inside the muscles, where it will be absorbed very quickly. (2) A large amount should be injected to lift both the fascia and the muscle, which requires more than 1–2 cc of filler. (3) The middle temporal vein, which runs horizontally at the temporal fossa under the superficial layer of the deep temporal fascia and is connected to the superficial temporal vein, should be avoided to prevent serious complications. The middle temporal vein is known to be located 23.5 mm (15.7–33.6 mm) above the jugale of the zygomatic arch and 18.5 mm (12.5–23.5 mm) above the zygion, one fingerbreadth above the zygomatic arch (Fig. 4.40). (4) According to a recent paper, there was a case report of penetration of the temporal bone during a needle injection. It is difficult to perforate the deep temporal fascia using a cannula; thus, a needle should be used to make deep injections. The authors prefer to inject into the

subcutaneous layer rather than deeply for the reasons described previously (Fig. 4.41). An injection using Koh's expanding technique (Fig. 4.29) is also useful in the temple area.

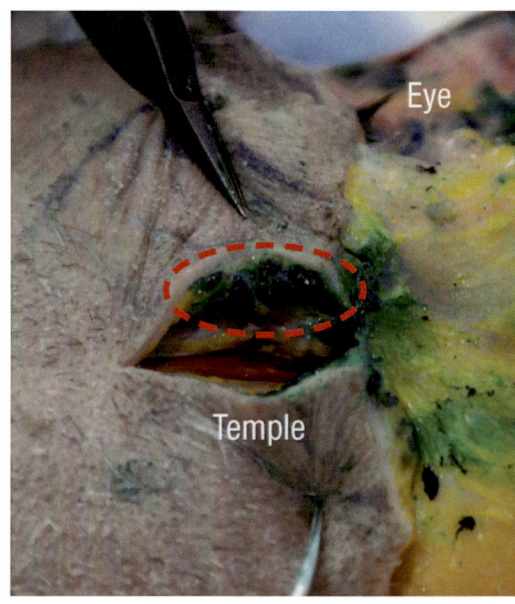

Fig. 4.41 Cadaveric dissection of a temple area injection. Blue-dyed filler is visible. Below the filler, multiple layers of temple are visible. The subcutaneous layer is relatively safe and requires less filler than deep injections

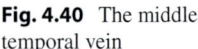

Fig. 4.40 The middle temporal vein

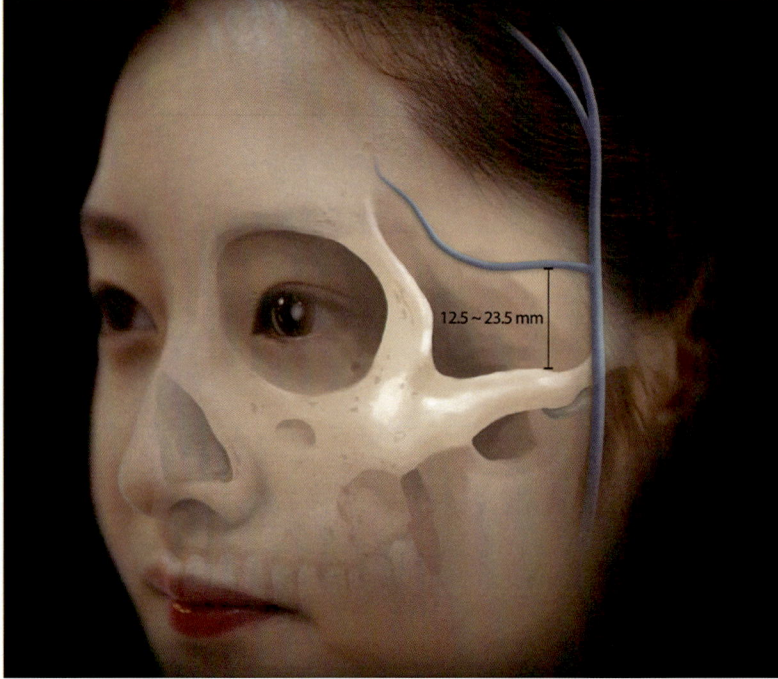

References

1. Ha RY, Nojima K, Adams WP Jr, Brown SA. Analysis of facial skin thickness: defining the relative thickness index. Plast Reconstr Surg. 2005;115(6):1769–73.
2. Lee W, Oh W, Hong GW, Kim JS, Yang EJ. Novel technique of filler injection in the temple area using the vein detection device. J Plast Reconstr Aesthet Surg. 2019;72:335–54.

Further Reading

1. Aulagnier J, Hoc C, Mathieu E, Dreyfus JF, Fischler M, Le Guen M. Efficacy of AccuVein to facilitate peripheral intravenous placement in adults presenting to an emergency department: a randomized clinical trial. Acad Emerg Med. 2014;21(8):858–63.
2. Breithaupt AD, Jones DH, Braz A, Narins R, Weinkle S. Anatomical basis for safe and effective volumization of the temple. Dermatol Surg. 2015;41(Suppl 1):S278–83.
3. Cong LY, Phothong W, Lee SH, Wanitphakdeedecha R, Koh I, Tansatit T, et al. Topographic analysis of the supratrochlear artery and the supraorbital artery: implication for improving the safety of forehead augmentation. Plast Reconstr Surg. 2017;139(3):620e–7e.
4. Davidge KM, van Furth WR, Agur A, Cusimano M. Naming the soft tissue layers of the temporoparietal region: unifying anatomic terminology across surgical disciplines. Neurosurgery. 2010;67(3 Suppl Operative):ons120–9; discussion ons9–30.
5. Erdogmus S, Govsa F. Anatomy of the supraorbital region and the evaluation of it for the reconstruction of facial defects. J Craniofac Surg. 2007;18(1):104–12.
6. Huang RL, Xie Y, Wang W, Herrler T, Zhou J, Zhao P, et al. Anatomical study of temporal fat compartments and its clinical application for temporal fat grafting. Aesthet Surg J. 2017;37(8):855–62.
7. Jung W, Youn KH, Won SY, Park JT, Hu KS, Kim HJ. Clinical implications of the middle temporal vein with regard to temporal fossa augmentation. Dermatol Surg. 2014;40(6):618–23.
8. O'Brien JX, Ashton MW, Rozen WM, Ross R, Mendelson BC. New perspectives on the surgical anatomy and nomenclature of the temporal region: literature review and dissection study. Plast Reconstr Surg. 2013;132(3):461e–3e.
9. Pessa JE, Kenkel JM, Heldermon CD. Periorbital and temporal anatomy, "Targeted Fat Grafting," and how a novel circulatory system in human peripheral nerves and brain may help avoid nerve injury and blindness during routine facial augmentation. Aesthet Surg J. 2017;37(8):969–73.
10. Saban Y, Andretto Amodeo C, Bouaziz D, Polselli R. Nasal arterial vasculature: medical and surgical applications. Arch Facial Plast Surg. 2012;14(6):429–36.
11. Scheuer JF 3rd, Sieber DA, Pezeshk RA, Campbell CF, Gassman AA, Rohrich RJ. Anatomy of the facial danger zones: maximizing safety during soft-tissue filler injections. Plast Reconstr Surg. 2017;139(1):50e–8e.
12. Wong CH, Hsieh MK, Mendelson B. The tear trough ligament: anatomical basis for the tear trough deformity. Plast Reconstr Surg. 2012;129(6):1392–402.

Skin Necrosis of Filler Injections

5

Skin necrosis after filler injection is quite a confusing experience for patients, while clinicians feel terrible having delivered what they assumed was a safe procedure. Consequences can even include permanent scarring.

Surprisingly, skin necrosis usually occurs when experienced rather than novice doctors perform filler injections since novice doctors tend to inject filler very carefully, while experienced doctors tend to increase the filler amount and inject it into multiple regions. Sometimes experienced doctors make the mistake of developing their own injection method without scientific evidence and considering filler injections an easy procedure. Thus, evidence-based education about skin necrosis is needed.

In this chapter, we will describe the mechanism, classification, diagnosis, and treatment of filler-induced skin necrosis.

5.1 Skin Necrosis Definition and Mechanism

5.1.1 Skin Necrosis Definition

Necrosis, defined as irreversible tissue damage followed by ischemic changes, occurs due to a break in the normal defense mechanism by ischemia-induced loss of tissue viability. In case of infection, extensive tissue can be destroyed by infectious necrosis.

Necrosis starts in the setting of a reduced vascular supply due to a direct embolism or compression by adjacent pressure. Filler injection-induced necrosis usually develops due to increased pressure rather than the direct needle puncture of a vessel.

Risk factors of necrosis are as follows:

- More superficial filler injection
- Thicker skin
- Harder skin
- Tighter skin
- Larger filler amount
- Greater swelling
- Small needle diameter

5.1.2 Mechanism

The vascular network becomes thinner and tighter as it approaches the dermal layer (Fig. 5.1). The dermis is harder and tighter than the deeper subcutaneous layer, so superficial injections increase the risk of vascular compression. Pressure also increases when a larger amount of filler is injected or tissue swelling develops.

The most common misunderstanding is that using a smaller-diameter needle is safer. According to Bernoulli's law, when a small-diameter needle is used, the injection pressure should be higher. While using a small-diameter needle, the injector feels greater viscosity and injects the filler with greater force. A smaller needle tip is also more likely to puncture a vessel and create an embolism; therefore, such needles are more dangerous than larger-diameter needles (Table 5.1).

© Springer Nature Singapore Pte Ltd. 2019
I. S. Koh, W. Lee, *Filler Complications*, https://doi.org/10.1007/978-981-13-6639-0_5

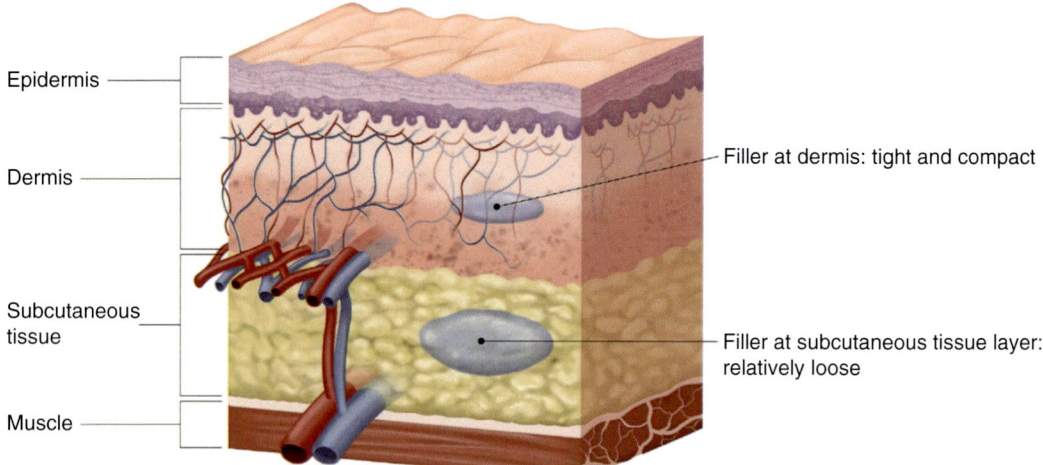

Epidermis

Dermis

Filler at dermis: tight and compact

Subcutaneous tissue

Filler at subcutaneous tissue layer: relatively loose

Muscle

Fig. 5.1 Cross-sectional schematic of the skin. The dermis is a very tight and compact structure compared to the subcutaneous tissue layer

Table 5.1 Risk factors of intravascular embolism

Increase risk of intravascular embolism	Small needle diameter (<27G)
	High-pressure injection
	Compression after bleeding
	Highly vascular region

Sudden swelling during an injection is likely indicative of bleeding. Compression is commonly used to treat such cases, but when filler is injected, compression could create an embolism and thus should not be done. Bleeding is a sign that the vessels are damaged and blood is extravasating. With compression, injected filler could be pushed into the vessel. When signs of bleeding are seen, it is best to stop the injection, remove the needle, and wait until the bleeding stops.

5.2 Classification of Skin Necrosis

Skin necrosis can be classified into localized and extended types. Localized necrosis develops at the injection site, whereas extended necrosis extends to the vascular territory (Fig. 5.2). The most severe complications of extended necrosis are blindness and cerebral infarction.

5.3 Localized Skin Necrosis

The dermal plexus is a small vascular network system located at the dermis or hypodermis. When filler is injected into this area, it is likely to compress the vessels and lead to skin necrosis because the tissue is unable to disperse the pressure. Interruptions in the circulation can also cause blanching. This blanching ischemia finishes within 30 minutes, and the localized change leads to a dark pinkish appearance and development of a pustule within 48 hours. Thereafter, infectious necrosis is likely to develop.

Mild vascular compression showing a small pustule and pinkish color might not require treatment. However, when compression is severe, the skin's color changes to a dark red wine color, and a pustule develops at each sebaceous gland. Pustules are likely connected to each other at the subcutaneous layer like underground water, and extensive infectious necrosis occurs. Tissue necrosis gradually develops and ultimately resolves as a depressive scar. If not treated properly, exudates changes to hard scabs that cover the necrotic surface. When a thick scab is formed, the infection progresses further, leading to further destruction of the subcutaneous tissue. An understanding of its pathophysiology is needed to determine the proper treatment (Figs. 5.3 and 5.4).

Fig. 5.2 Pathophysiology of skin necrosis induced by vascular obstruction

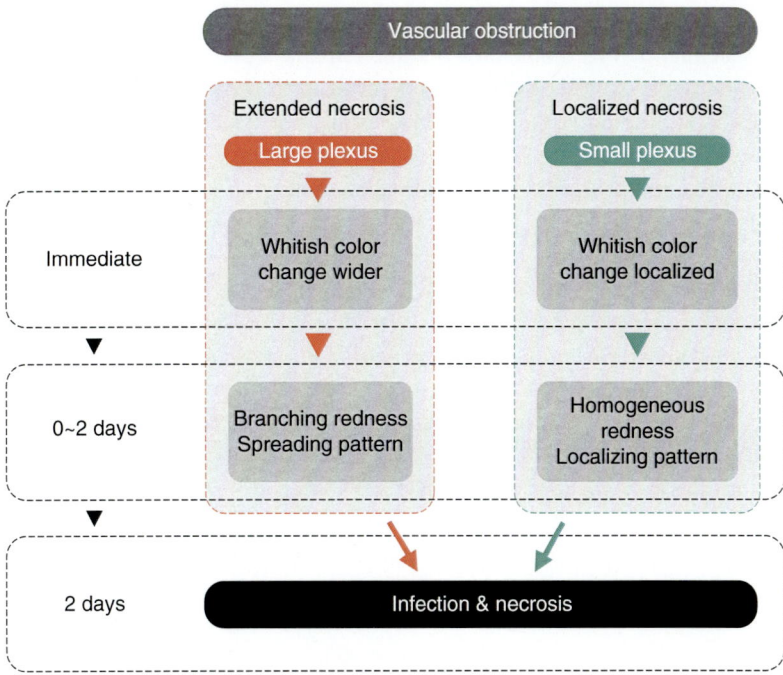

Fig. 5.3 Relatively mild case of localized skin necrosis. Photograph of a patient's nose 3 days after the injection of the hyaluronic acid filler. The untreated area looks severe because of the numerous visible pustules. However, the amount of pus was small, the skin is pinkish, and only mild inflammation is visible, so a good prognosis is expected

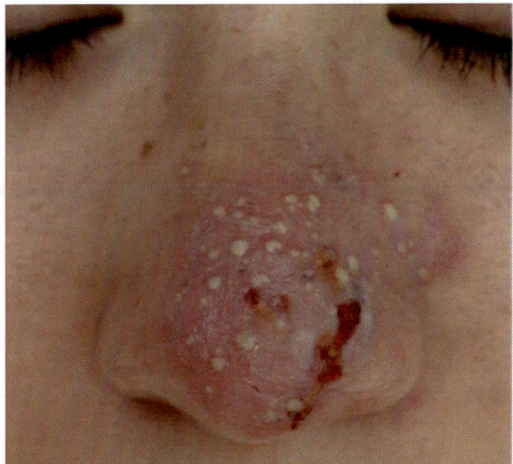

Fig. 5.4 Severe case of localized skin necrosis. Photograph of a patient's nose 4 days after the injection of the permanent filler. Multiple damaged regions are visible. The pus is widespread and the skin has developed a red wine color. The most damaged region is black, indicating necrosis. The predicted prognosis is poor

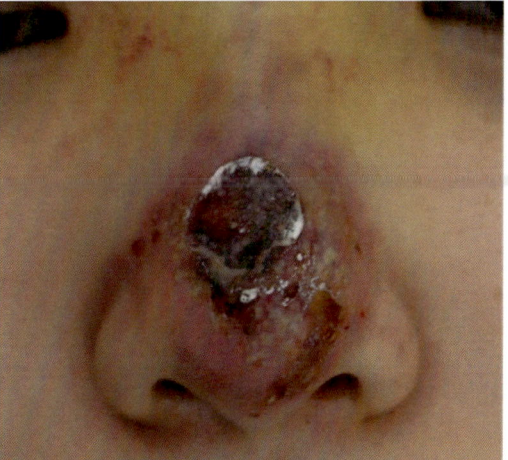

5.3.1 Treatment

5.3.1.1 Decompression

Blanching after a filler injection should immediately be treated with decompression. When hyaluronic acid filler is injected, a high dose is needed to dissolve the filler. We prefer to inject one vial (1500 IU) of hyaluronidase mixed with 1–1.5 mL of normal saline and massage gently. There are no guidelines for hyaluronidase injections, but we prefer to use a high dose. If any filler remains undissolved, more hyaluronidase should be injected, but since the tissue is very friable due to ischemia, it is recommended that the remaining filler be dissolved at once. When permanent or calcium filler remains undissolved, it must be removed as soon as possible using negative pressure with large-diameter (18G) needle aspiration.

It is important to call the patient 1 day after injection to check for any color change or specific symptoms. A photograph of the patient should be checked if unusual progress is seen. Patients are likely to come to the clinic after the second day with complications because of pustules. Thus, if decompression is performed as soon as possible, patient status should be checked 1 day later.

Pustules usually develop within 2 days after the injection, so patients tend to visit the clinic themselves. Therefore, it is very important to check 1 day after the injection. Patients who tend to describe their symptoms as not severe should be evaluated using a photograph or in person.

5.3.1.2 Dressing (Figs. 5.5 and 5.6)

5.3.1.3 Pustule Removal
Pustules likely develop if decompression is not performed or vessels are severely compressed within 48 hours. More aggressive treatment should be performed when pustules develop before 48 hours because such cases can progress to severe necrosis.

Pustules should be removed gently because the area including the nose and maxilla is considered the danger triangle of the face due to venous communication between the facial vein and the cavernous sinus. A retrograde infection can spread to the brain, causing cavernous sinus thrombosis or meningitis.

The appropriate drainage of pustules can be encouraged by the use of oral medication.

Pustules are likely to spread within 48–72 hours, reduce 4 days after, and disappear within 6 days after the injection. Thus, pustule removal should be performed twice daily at 2–4 days after the injection. And it is important to prevent infection whenever possible and prevent depressed scar formation. After the acute infection stage, small pustules may appear but are easily cured.

5.3.1.4 Closed Wet Dressing
Necrotic tissue rapidly loses water and becomes covered by scabs. Pus under the thick scab tends to destroy the subcutaneous layer and create a depressed scar. Thus, a dressing should be applied to prevent scab formation. A wet dressing substitutes for the scab. We initially remove the pus and exudate, clean the wound, apply an antiseptic, and cover the wound with Vaseline gauze. The occlusive dressing is used until the pustules disappear. Hydrocolloid products are not recommended because they are best used when dressing changes are not required.

It is important that the skin not become detached during dressing changes, so we must be careful when removing the Vaseline gauze. Gentle removal and the use of a watery antiseptic are recommended. Even if the damaged skin is unviable, it is still useful as a biological dressing. Comparison of the removed skin and unremoved skin groups revealed that the unremoved group had much better results. Use of the Vaseline gauze dressing also minimizes skin defects (Figs. 5.6 and 5.7).

5.3.1.5 Treatment After Acute Stage
After the acute stage, which should be treated as soon as possible, careful observation and education is needed to minimize sequelae. When providing aggressive and appropriate treatment, a complete cure can be accomplished without sequelae. Minor sequelae may include dermatitis or small pustules. Post-inflammatory hyperpigmentation occurs easily and is difficult to treat, so close observation and education are needed. Hyperpigmentation has no specific treatment other than UV protection for 6 months. Severe sequelae such as contracture, skin defect, and a depressive scar could occur when inappropriate treatment is provided and then require secondary treatment such as cell therapy.

5.3.1.6 Misunderstanding Treatment
Filler injections have been proposed as groundbreaking treatments, but many of them are not scientifically proven.

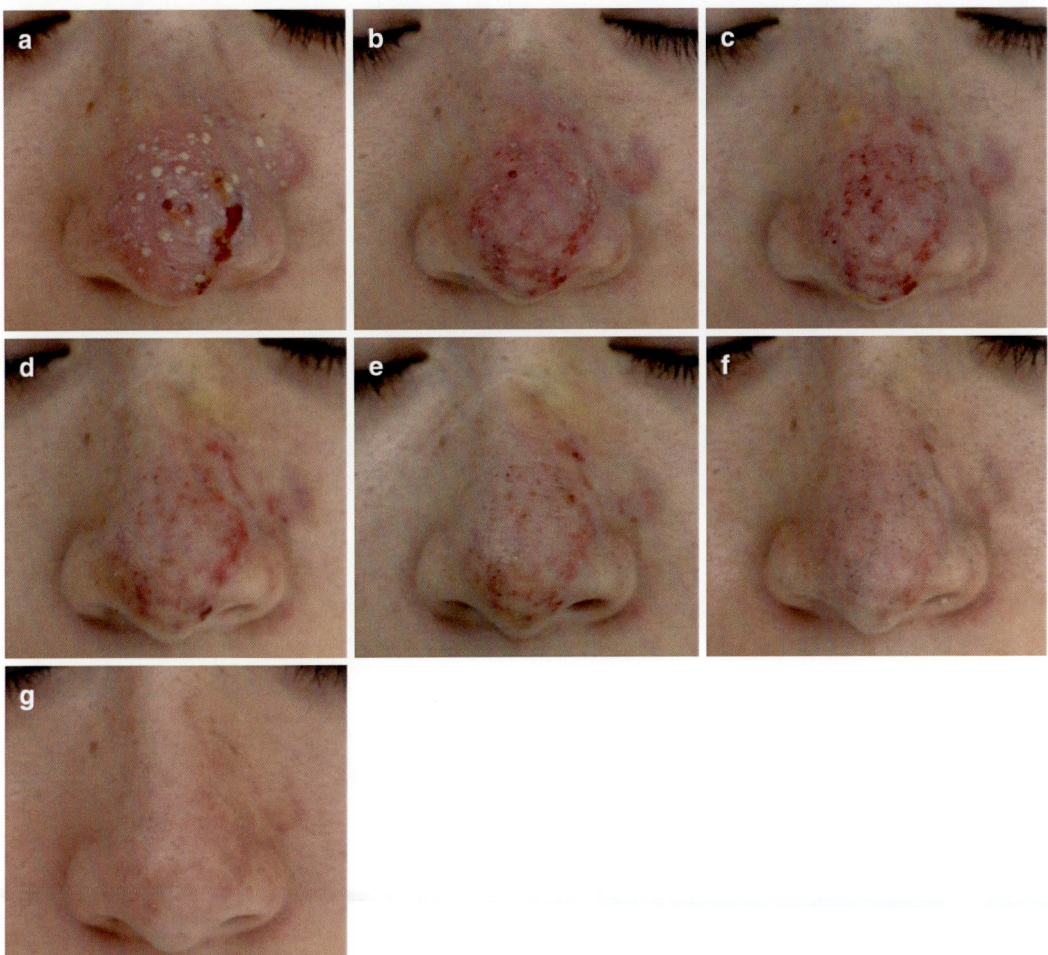

Fig. 5.5 Treatment progress of a mild case of localized skin necrosis. A case of localized skin necrosis that developed after the injection of the hyaluronic acid filler was eradicated after appropriate treatment. (**a**) Photograph of a patient's nose 3 days after filler injection. The area looks severely injured due to the presence of many pustules. (**b**) The patient's nose 4 days after filler injection and before the first treatment. Pustules are likely to develop in 2–4 days and should be removed at least twice daily. (**c**) The patient's nose 4 days after filler injection and before the second treatment. The pustules are removed twice daily and their number decreases. (**d**) The patient's nose 5 days after filler injection. When pustules are no longer present, the dressings are reduced to once a day to enable skin regeneration. (**e**) The patient's nose 6 days after filler injection. An occlusive wet dressing is applied to prevent drying of the area. (**f**) The patient's nose 8 days after filler injection. The dressings are removed once the tissues are healthy enough. The recovered tissues are relatively sensitive to UV light, so patients should be warned about post-inflammatory hyperpigmentation. (**g**) The patient's nose 3 weeks after filler injection showing complete healing. Mild problems such as dermatitis might occur, so the patient should be reevaluated regularly

Hyperbaric oxygen therapy has been proposed as a good treatment. However, problems occur when only hyperbaric oxygen therapy is used. We have multiple experiences with filler complications and bad prognosis in patients who were treated with only hyperbaric oxygen therapy. Hyperbaric oxygen therapy should be an adjuvant treatment. The most important treatments are pustule removal, decompression, and occlusive dressings (Fig. 5.8).

Another proposed treatment is stem cell therapy, which will be groundbreaking in many medical fields. However, it is not useful for treating acute ischemic necrosis. Stem

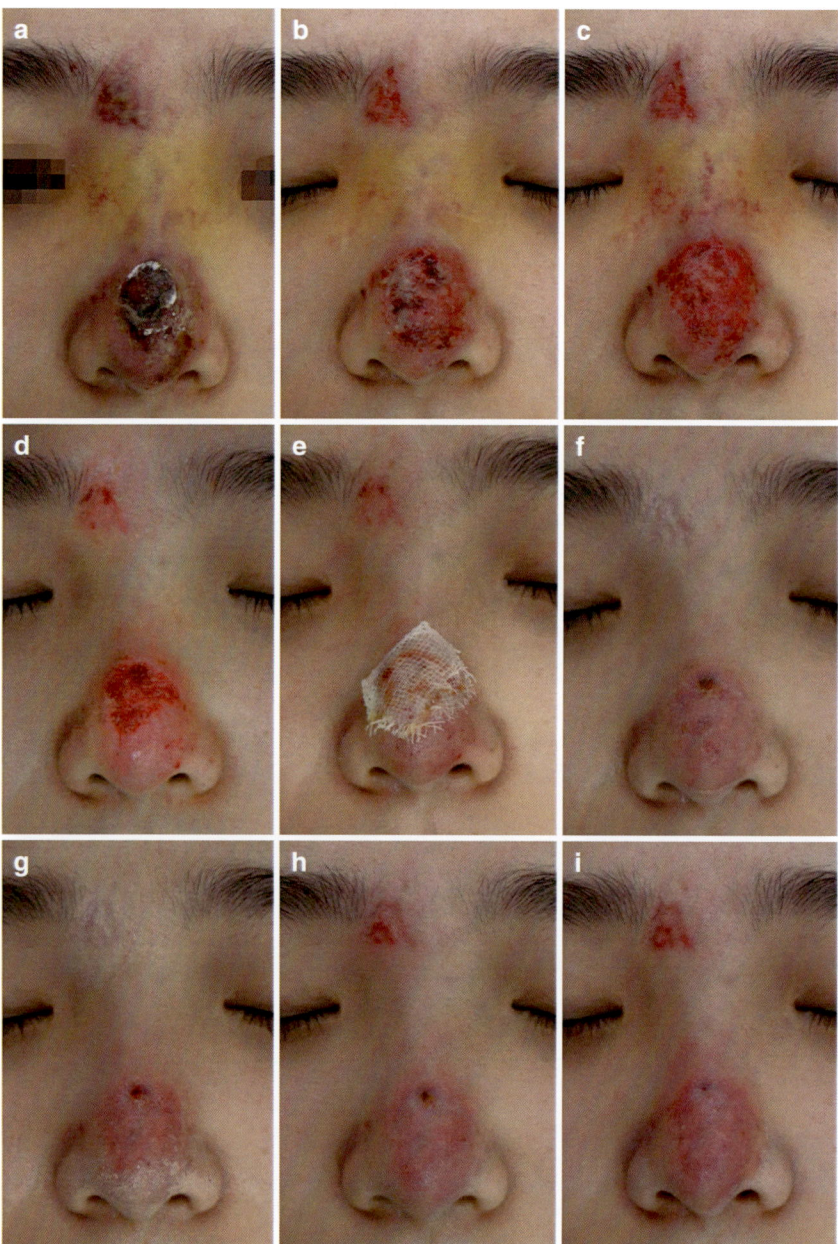

Fig. 5.6 Treatment progress of severe case of localized skin necrosis. Injection of the permanent filler requires observation for 1 year. (**a**) At 4 days after the injection, severe skin necrosis appeared and a thick scab formed. Some extensive skin necrosis of the dorsal nasal artery and supratrochlear artery territories was also noted. Immediate debridement was performed and an occlusive dressing was applied. (**b**) The area 5 days after injection. Necrotic tissues are still visible in the most damaged region. (**c**) The area 5 days after injection required further debridement. (**d**) The area 13 days after injection. The severely damaged region shows loss of the subcutaneous layer, but the surrounding tissues are relatively intact. (**e**) The area 15 days after injection. Vaseline gauze was applied to encourage re-epithelialization. By this time, adjuvant wound healing products such as epidermal growth factor and polydeoxyribonucleotides could be applied. (**f**) The area 20 days after injection. Most of the region is covered with friable tissues. (**g**) The area 21 days after injection. (**h**) The area 25 days after injection. (**i**) The area 27 days after injection. (**j**) The area 29 days after injection. (**k**) The area 45 days after injection. (**l**) The area 2 months after injection. New vessels (angiogenesis) are visible in the granulation tissue. (**m**) The area 3 months after injection. Further angiogenesis is noted. (**n**) The area 4 months after injection. The skin is red due to continued angiogenesis. (**o**) The area 6 months after injection shows that the skin has turned pinkish. (**p**) The area 9 months after injection showing a diminished pink color of the skin. (**q**) The area 1 year after injection showing an almost normalized skin color. Other treatments can be considered for the depressed scar

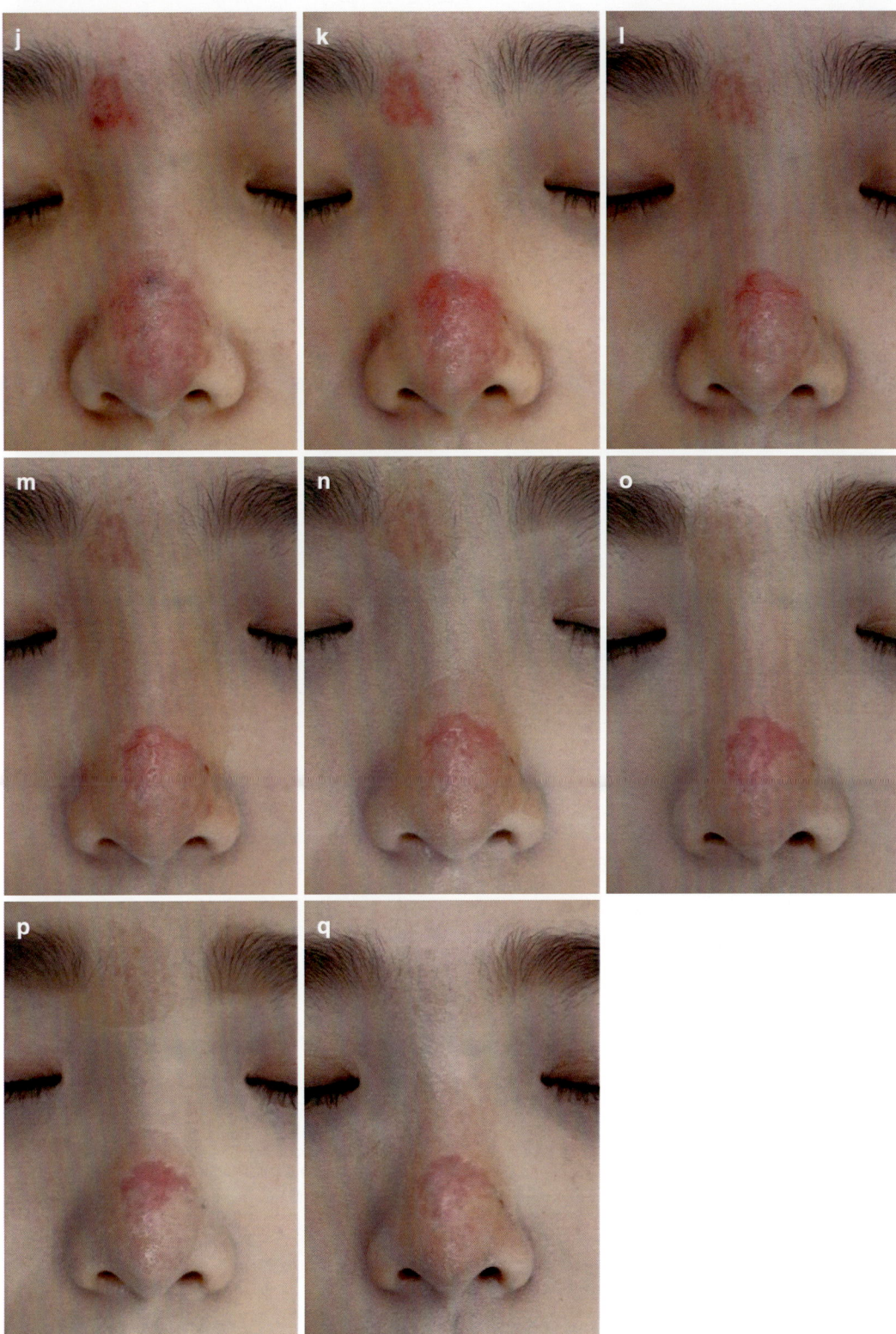

Fig. 5.6 (continued)

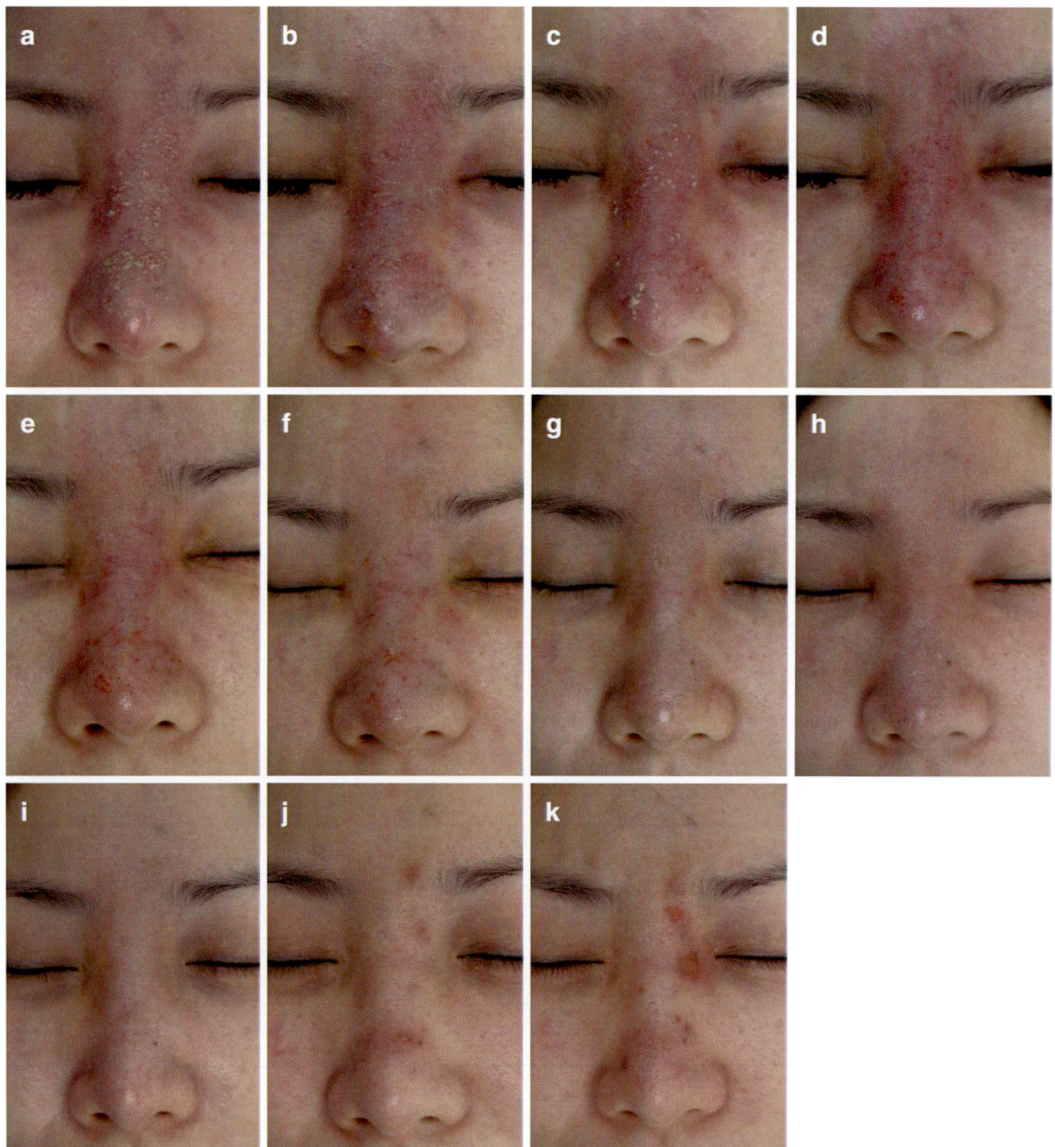

Fig. 5.7 Treatment progress of a severe case of localized skin necrosis. Localized severe skin necrosis developed 36 hours after the injection of the hyaluronic acid filler into the nose. (**a**) The area 36 hours after the injection. Multiple pustules appeared prior to 36 hours, indicating that aggressive treatment is needed for severely compromised vascularity. (**b**) The area 2 days after the injection after the first treatment and before the second treatment. The pustules were removed during the first treatment but recurred 4 hours later. Repeated removal is very important in cases of severely compromised vascularity. (**c**) The area 3 days after the injection and before the second treatment. Multiple pustules are visible. (**d**) The area 3 days after the injection and after the second treatment. (**e**) The area 4 days after the injection. Since pustules are not visible, a wet dressing was applied once a day. (**f**) The area 5 days after the injection. Since the swelling was reduced and the infectious signs decreased, hyaluronidase was used to dissolve the hyaluronic acid filler. (**g**) The area 7 days after the injection. Since the swelling was reduced and infectious signs had decreased, hyaluronidase was used to dissolve the hyaluronic acid filler. (**h**) The area 8 days after the injection. Minimal swelling occurred. (**i**) The area 13 days after the injection. The patient's condition was almost recovered. (**j**) The area 27 days after the injection. Small pustules and a slight color change are visible. Such patients should be observed for at least 6 months. (**k**) The area 32 days after the injection showing that the patient's symptoms are aggravated

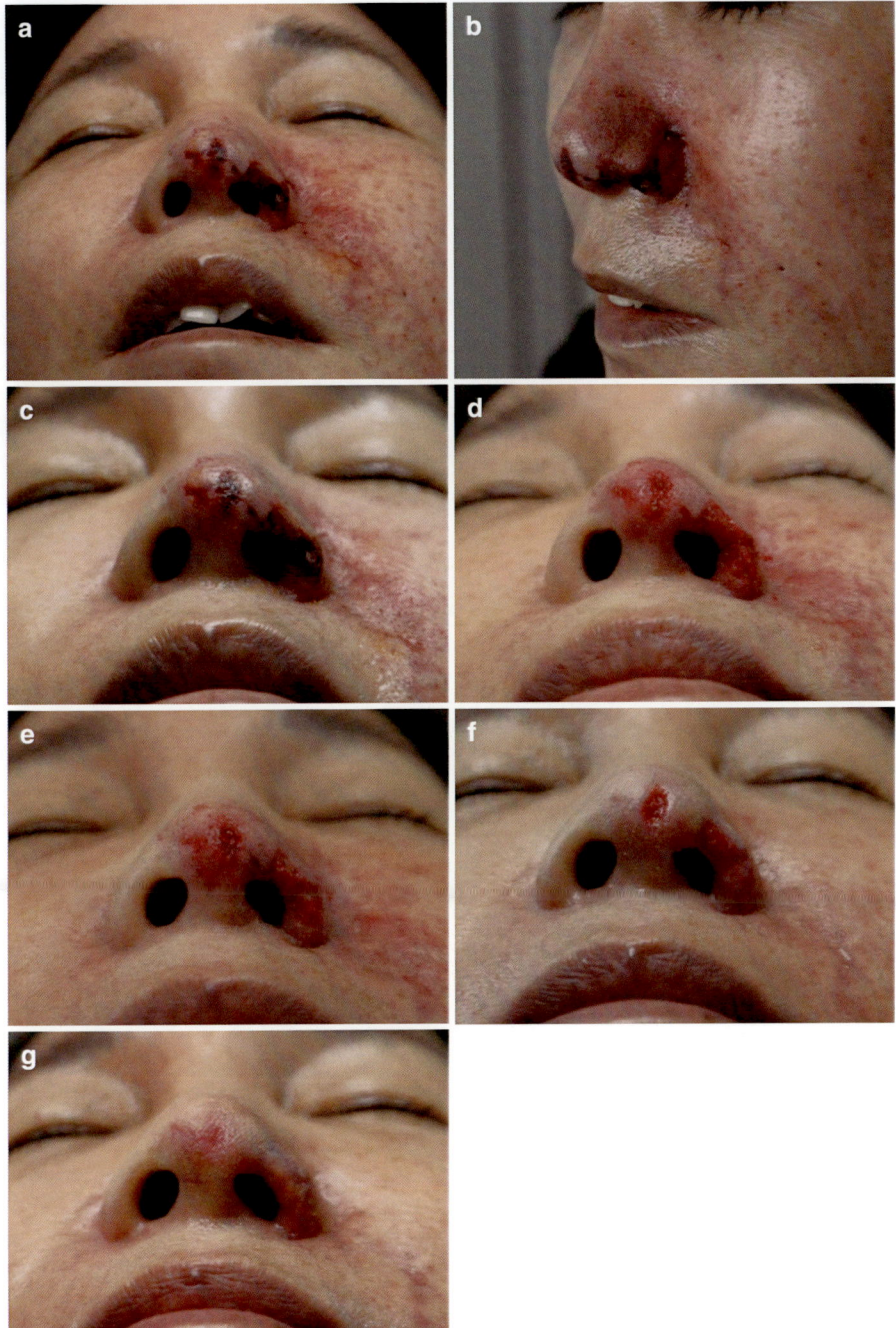

Fig. 5.8 Extensive skin necrosis case treated with only hyperbaric oxygen and vasodilation. Extensive skin necrosis caused by the injection of the hyaluronic acid filler into the nasolabial fold and lateral nasal artery territories. The wound dried due to the use of only hyperbaric oxygen therapy. The skin was recovered by debridement, and closed wet dressings were used to promote healing. (a) Pretreatment image taken 11 days after the injection of a hyaluronic acid filler into the nasolabial fold. The wound was covered with scabs and unhealthy. (b) Pretreatment image. (c) Pretreatment image (worm's-eye view). (d) Post-debridement image. (e) The area 1 day after treatment. Healthy viable tissues are visible. (f) The area 9 days after treatment. Reepithelialization is visible. (g) The area 14 days after treatment. The skin defect has been covered with epithelium. (h) Example of a closed wet dressing. Antiseptic use, scab removal, and Vaseline gauze application to keep the wound wet are important. (i) Example of closed wet dressing. Both the necrotized area and the vascular compromised area should be covered

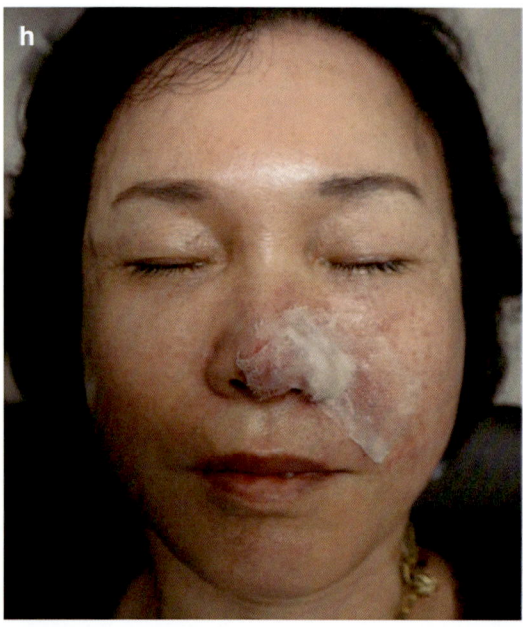
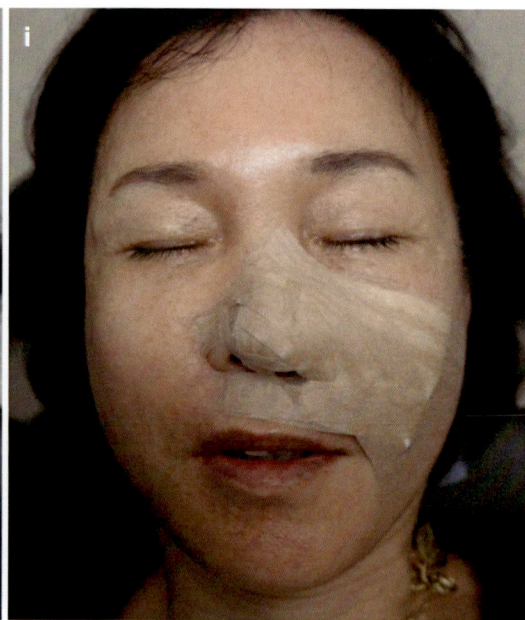

Fig. 5.8 (continued)

cell therapy might be applied 4–5 days after the pustules have cleared.

A skin graft is useful for treating skin defects. However, a skin graft should never be performed for a nose defect because the nose has distinctly thick skin and a texture that differs from other areas. The use of careful dressings that preserve the tissue and promote reepithelialization could lead to better final results (Fig. 5.6).

In the treatment of necrotic tissue, occlusive dressings should be used instead of open dressings (Fig. 5.9). Open dressings dry the wound and lead to scab formation. During the acute stage, hydrocolloid products should not be used because the wound exudate should be properly removed.

Many treatments have been suggested, but they should be considered adjuvant therapy to encourage wound healing.

5.4   Extended Necrosis

Extended necrosis progresses as arborization of the vessel territories. Extensive necrosis occurs because of large vessel involvement and divided into proximal necrosis, that near the injection site, or distal necrosis, that far from the injection site.

5.4.1   Proximal Necrosis

This phenomenon is seen when larger-diameter vessels are compressed or occluded, rather than small-diameter vessels such as those in the subdermal plexus. Necrosis occurring along the vessel pathway resembles arborization (Figs. 5.1 and 5.2).

The most necrotized area is the vessel-affected region, and it spreads along the vascular territory of the area of proximal necrosis. Severe compression or thrombosis at the traumatized vessel and necrosis at that region is the cause. Proximal necrosis is usually combined with distal necrosis since thrombosis usually occurs. Thus, when extended necrosis is detected, the involved vessel must be identified and decompressed as soon as possible. If hyaluronic acid filler is used, a high concentration of hyaluronidase is recommended to dissolve it. If a calcium or permanent filler is used, a needle larger than 18G must be used for decom-

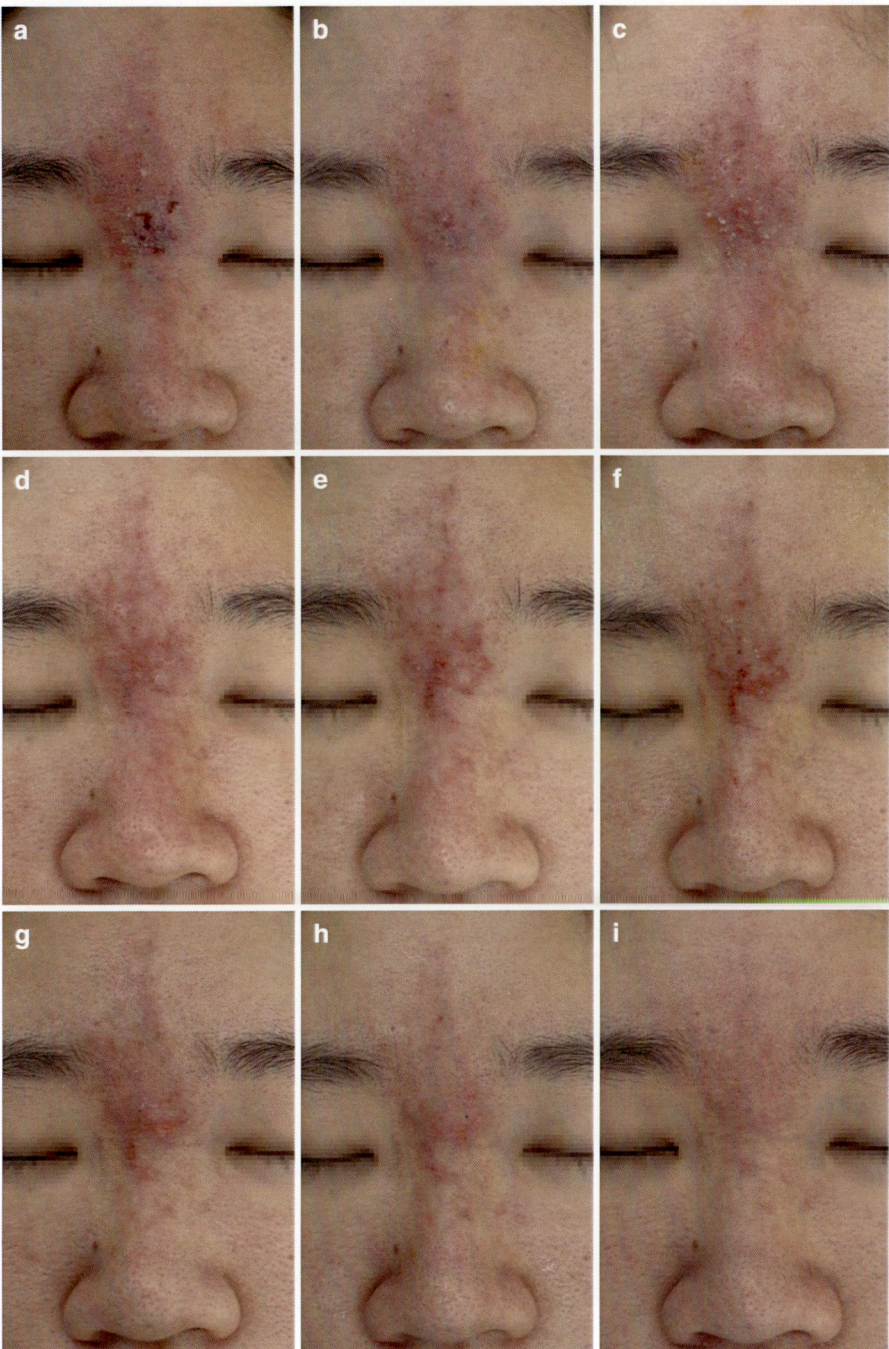

Fig. 5.9 Treatment progress of nasal root skin necrosis. Two days after the hyaluronic acid filler was injected into the dorsum of the nose, extensive necrosis became visible at the supratrochlear artery territory. (**a**) Two days after the injection, the supratrochlear artery territory is also involved. (**b**) Two days after the injection and the first treatment, the pustules have disappeared. (**c**) Three days after the injection, multiple pustules are visible. Twice-daily treatment is essential to manage the developing pustules. (**d**) Three days after the injection but before the second treatment. (**e**) Four days after the injection, pustules are no longer visible, so a once-daily dressing is used. (**f**) Five days after the injection, the wound has dried and aggravated due to observation by another doctor, who removed the occlusive dressing. This demonstrates the importance of a wet dressing. (**g**) Seven days after the injection. (**h**) Eight days after the injection. (**i**) Seventeen days after the injection, the area was almost healed with a minimal color change

pression. It is important to confirm which vessel is involved and then decompress it. The wound dressing should be the same as that used to treat localized necrosis (Figs. 5.10, 5.11, and 5.12).

These affected vessels include the lateral nasal artery, facial artery (Fig. 5.13), dorsal nasal artery (Fig. 5.14), supratrochlear artery (Fig. 5.15), and supraorbital artery (Fig. 5.16).

5.4.2 Distant Necrosis

The needle or cannula tip puncturing the vessel or the injection of filler into a torn vessel creates an embolism; in the most severe cases, blindness or cerebral infarction may occur.

In cases of distant necrosis, the most severe necrosis develops at the distant region including

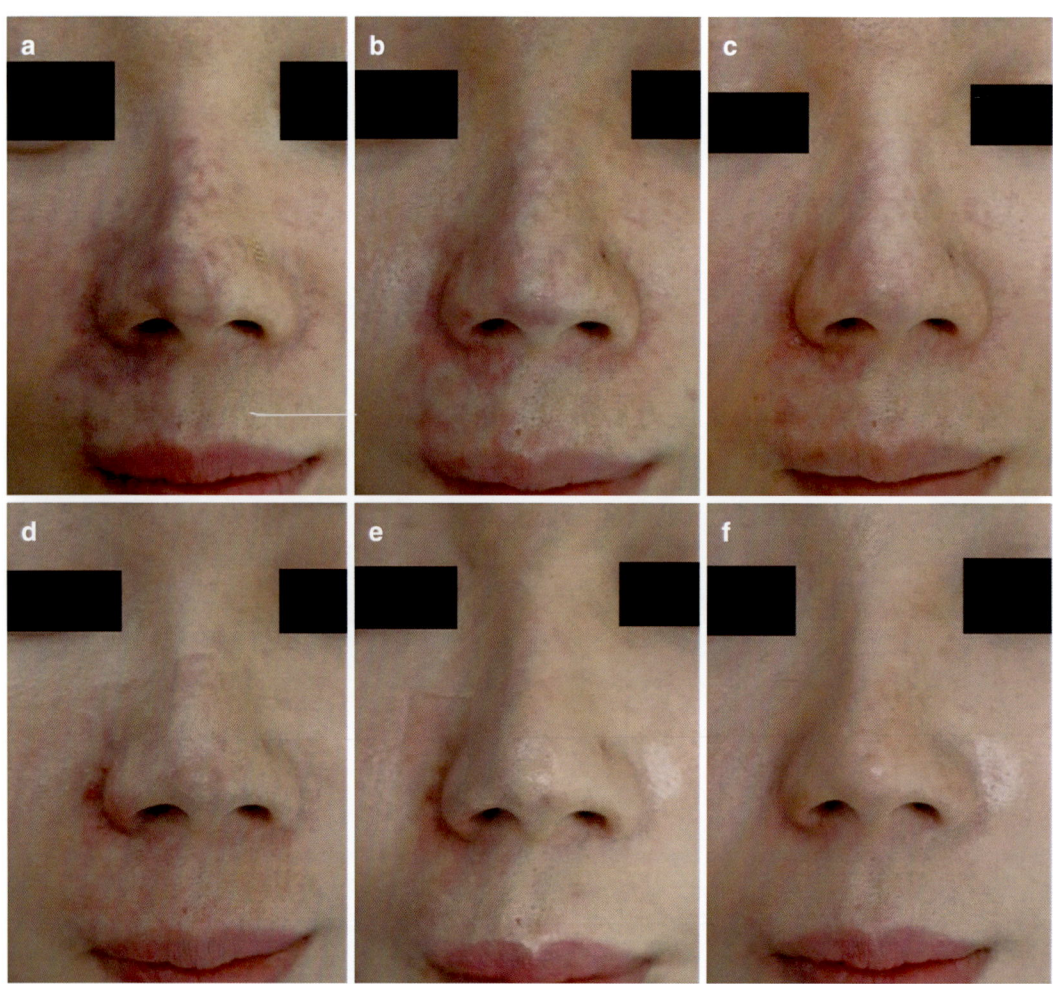

Fig. 5.10 Extensive necrosis after nasolabial fold correction. Extensive necrosis appeared after the injection of the hyaluronic acid filler into the nasolabial fold. The lateral nasal artery territory was involved, and hyaluronidase was immediately injected. Severe compression during the filler injection occurred, but it recovered within 1 week because of the early treatment. (**a**) The lateral nasal artery territories demonstrated ischemic changes after nasolabial fold correction. We injected hyaluronidase and transferred her to our clinic within 6 hours after the filler injection. The skin has changed color at the lateral nasal, superior labial, and dorsal nasal artery territories. (**b**) The area 1 day after the injection. Revascularization signs are visible. (**c**) The area 2 days after the injection. A few pustules are visible in the most severely affected area. (**d**) The area 4 days after the injection. (**e**) The area 7 days after the injection. Pustules are not visible and the skin color has recovered. (**f**) The area 2 months after the injection. The patient has healed completely without any sequelae

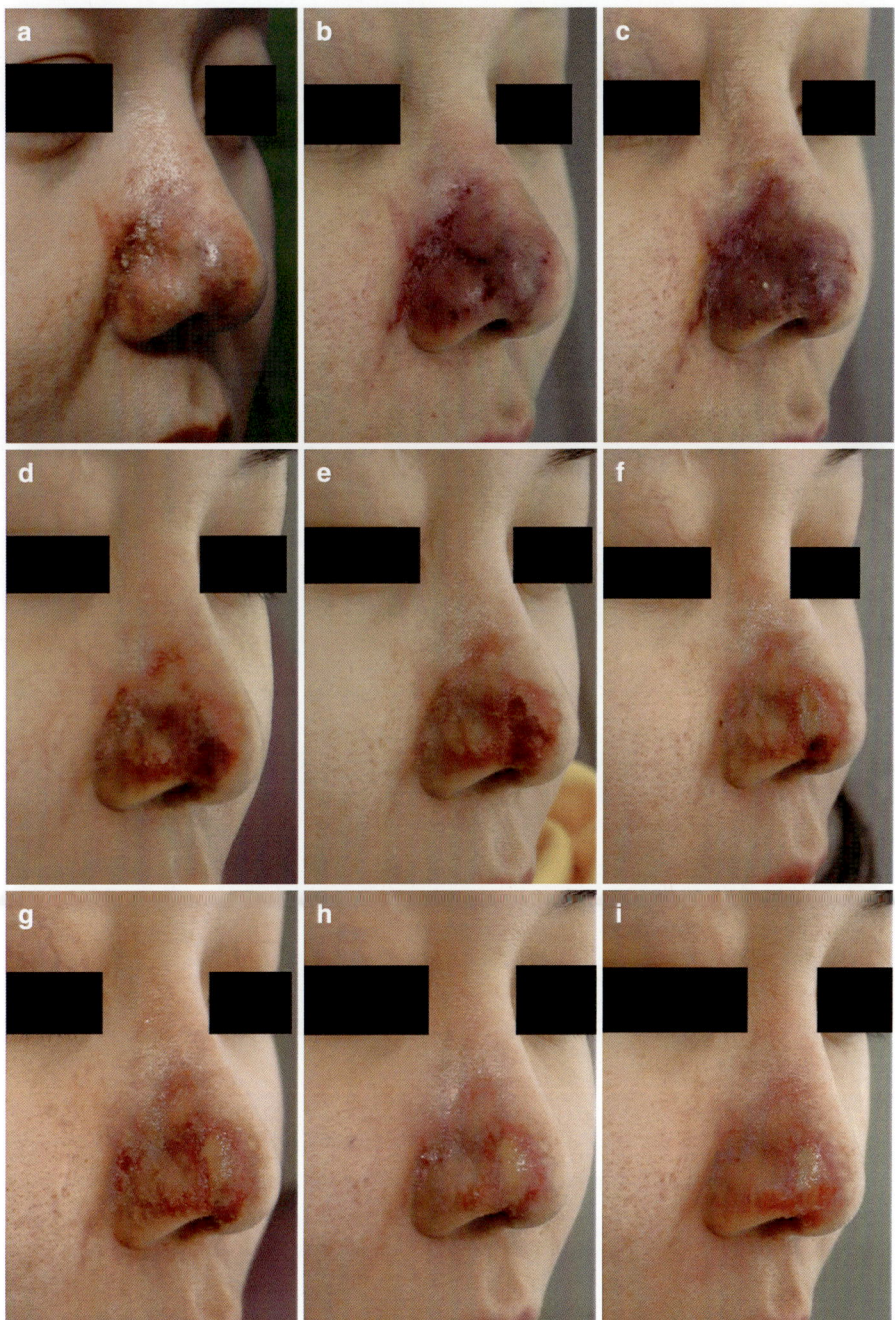

Fig. 5.11 Severe extensive necrosis after nasolabial fold correction. Three days after the injection of the hyaluronic acid filler. The progression of extensive necrosis is visible, indicating damage to the lateral nasal artery. The late treatment caused the long recovery time. (**a**) The area 3 days after the filler injection. Severe tissue damage is indicated by the dark wine color. (**b**) The pustules have disappeared. (**c**) The area 4 days after the filler injection. The skin gradually changed to necrotic tissue. (**d**) The area 7 days after the injection. More aggravated necrosis is visible. (**e**) The area 8 days after the injection. The most severe necrosis is seen at terminal territory of the lateral nasal artery. (**f**) The area 9 days after the injection. Eschar formation is visible at the nasal tip area. (**g**) The area 10 days after the injection. (**h**) The area 11 days after the injection. (**i**) The area 13 days after the injection. The yellowish necrotic tissues require removal. (**j**) The area 15 days after the injection and 2 days after debridement. (**k**) The area 22 days after the injection and 9 days after debridement with Vaseline gauze applied. (**l**) The area 24 days after the injection. Epithelialization is visible. (**m**) The area 29 days after the injection. Reduced skin defects are visible. (**n**) The area 5 weeks after the injection. Minimal hypertrophic scars are visible. (**o**) The area 4 months after the injection. The patient has recovered and the scar is unnoticeable

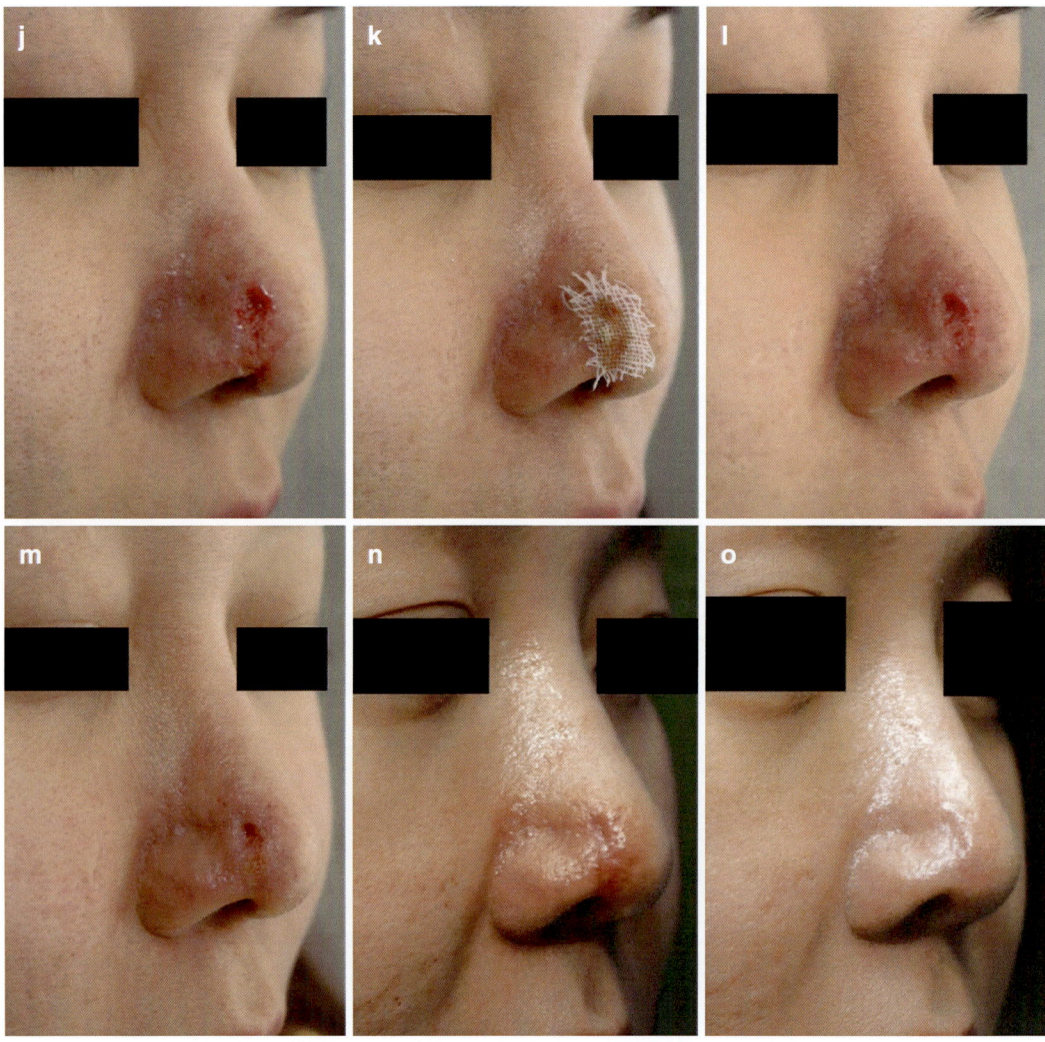

Fig. 5.11 (continued)

emboli occluding the vessel. Reactive hyperemia is not seen in the occluded vessel. Blood supply is likely increased due to the distant partial occlusion. This phenomenon can be seen in large-diameter vessels such as the facial artery and/or the superficial temporal artery (Figs. 5.17, 5.18, and 5.19).

Cases involving large filler embolisms are susceptible to proximal and distant necrosis. In this case, much more severe necrosis develops and needs more aggressive treatments.

In cases of distant necrosis, sufficient hyaluronidase should be injected into the filler-injected portion and the distant necrotic area.

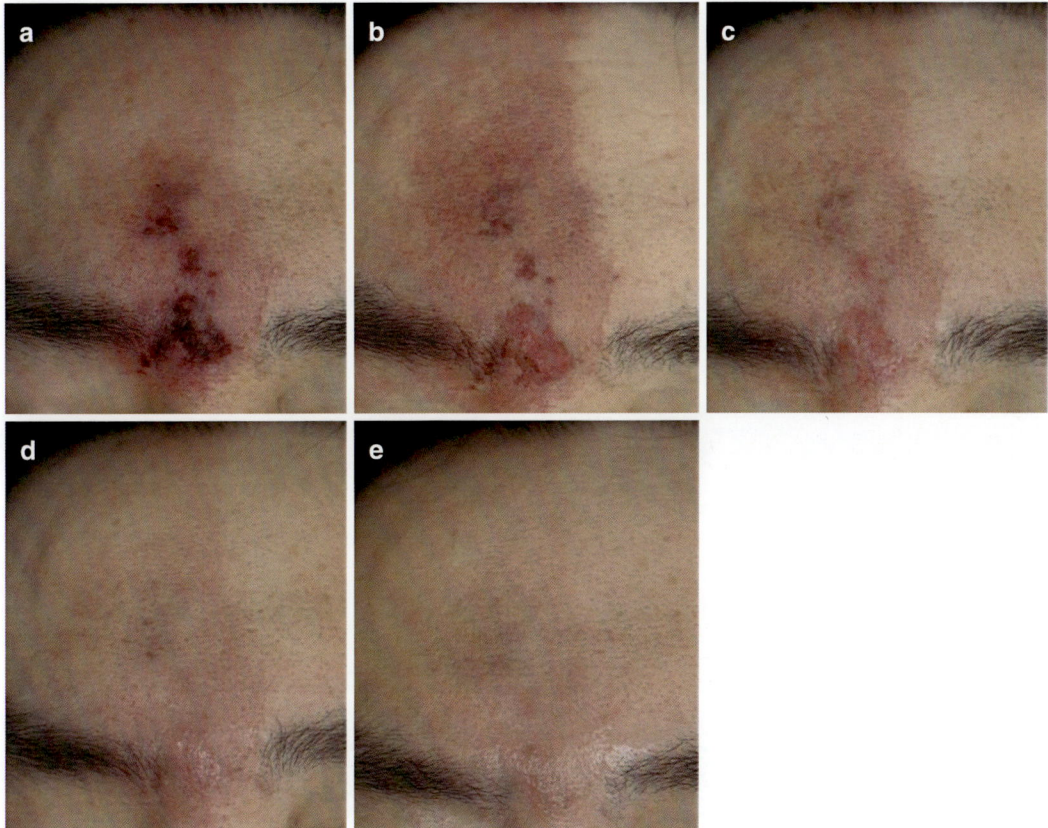

Fig. 5.12 Extensive necrosis after correction of a glabellar wrinkle. Extensive necrosis after the injection of the hyaluronic acid filler for the correction of a glabellar wrinkle. The supratrochlear artery territory was damaged. (**a**) The area 4 days after the injection. The supratrochlear artery territories are involved. The wound dried due to use of an open dressing. However, the surrounding tissues are pinkish and healthy, indicating a good prognosis. (**b**) The area 6 days after the injection. The dried necrotized tissues have been exfoliated. However, the dermal layer remains intact, so a depressed scar may not form, but the color of the supratrochlear territory indicates aggravation. (**c**) The area 8 days after the injection. The skin color has improved and epithelialization has developed. (**d**) The area 10 days after the injection. The patient has almost recovered. (**e**) The area 22 days after the injection. The patient had completely healed except for the glabella. This region healed within 3 months

However, if the filler was a permanent type, such as calcium filler or PCL filler, its removal is not recommended because it might harm unstable necrotic tissues; rather, it should be dressed.

To reduce this risk, we must use a needle larger than 23G and inject the filler gently with low pressure. Avoid injecting into the main vessel layer. When the vessel is ruptured, one should stop injecting filler and wait until the bleeding stops. It is possible that the filler could move into the ruptured vessel during compression to stop the bleeding. Blindness, one of the most serious complications, was described in Chap. 6.

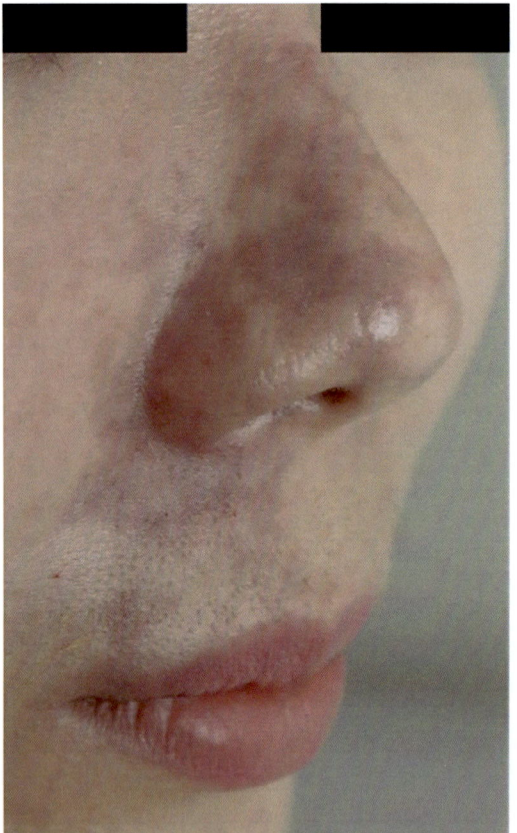

Fig. 5.13 Extensive necrosis of the lateral nasal artery. Extensive necrosis developed at the lateral nasal artery territory after nasolabial fold correction

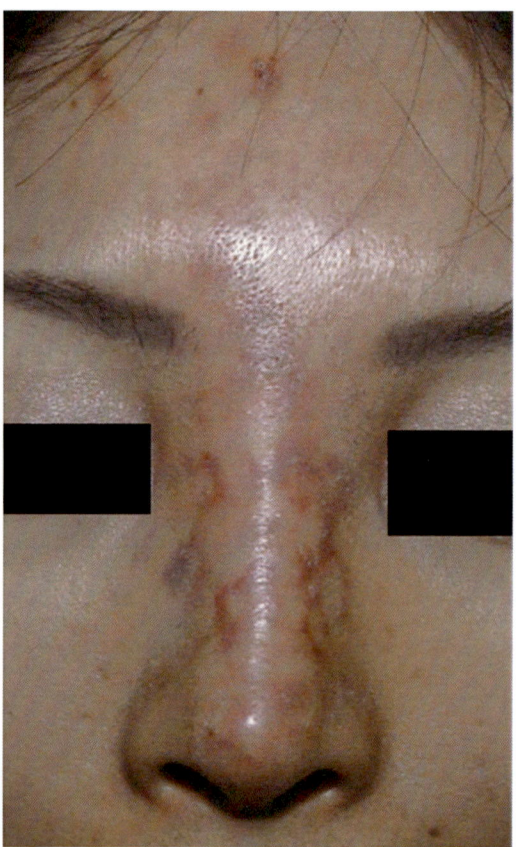

Fig. 5.14 Extensive necrosis of the dorsal nasal artery. Extensive necrosis developed at the dorsal nasal artery territory after nose filler augmentation. The supratrochlear artery territory was also affected

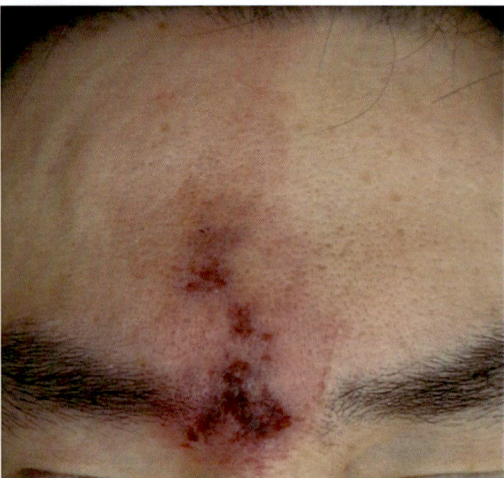

Fig. 5.15 Extensive necrosis of the supratrochlear artery. Extensive necrosis developed in the supratrochlear artery territory after glabellar wrinkle correction

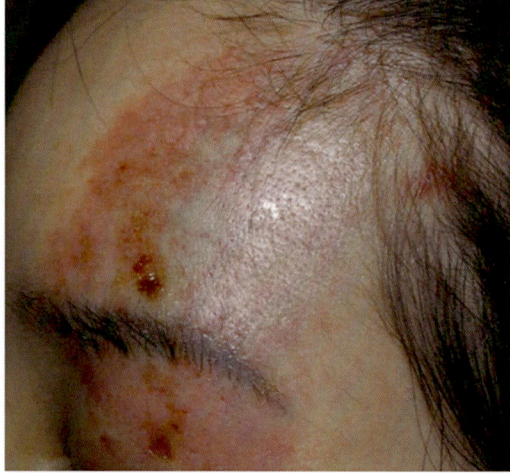

Fig. 5.16 Extensive necrosis of the supraorbital artery. Extensive necrosis developed in the supraorbital territory after forehead augmentation

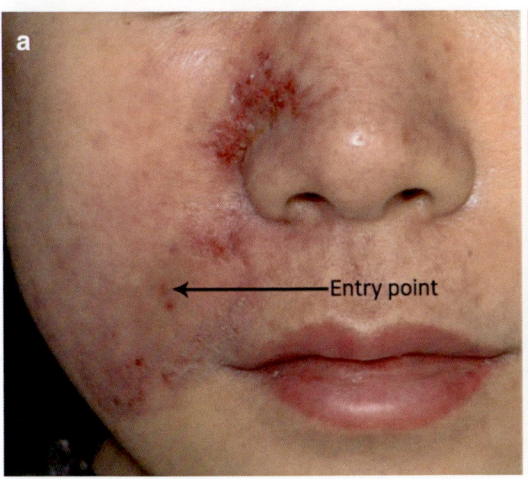
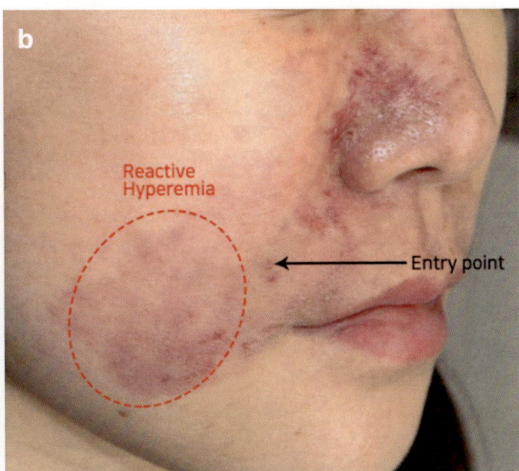

Fig. 5.17 Distant extensive necrosis after nasolabial fold correction. Distant extensive necrosis developed 4 days after the injection of the hyaluronic acid filler for nasolabial fold correction. (**a**) An embolism occurred in the right facial artery and lateral nasal artery distant territories, and the angular artery territory became necrotic. The most distant location from the entry point is the most necrotic. (**b**) Typical reactive hyperemia is observed before the entry point due to compensatory excessive circulation induced by the distant occlusion

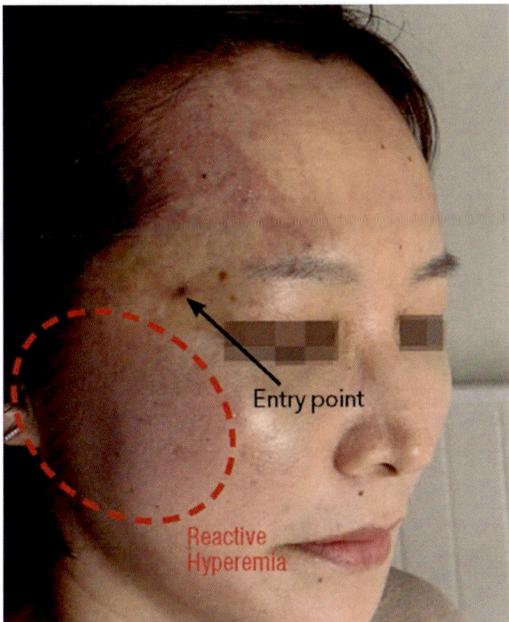

Fig. 5.18 Distant extensive skin necrosis and reactive hyperemia after filler injection into the temple area. Three days after the hyaluronic acid filler was injected into the temple area. An embolism occurred at the superficial temporal artery and skin necrosis developed in its territory. The supraorbital artery territory was not affected. Reactive hyperemia is visible before the entry point

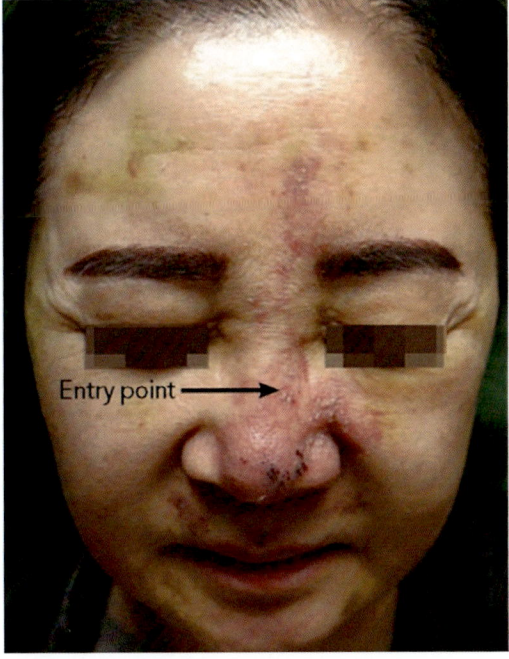

Fig. 5.19 Distant extensive necrosis. Four days after nose augmentation by the hyaluronic acid filler. An embolism caused necrosis and pustules at the nasal tip and affected the supratrochlear area

Further Reading

1. Lemperle G, Gauthier-Hazan N, Wolters M, Eisemann-Klein M, Zimmermann U, Duffy DM. Foreign body granulomas after all injectable dermal fillers: part 1. Possible causes. Plast Reconstr Surg. 2009;123(6):1842–63.
2. Ono S, Ogawa R, Hyakusoku H. Complications after polyacrylamide hydrogel injection for soft-tissue augmentation. Plast Reconstr Surg. 2010;126(4):1349–57.
3. Ozturk CN, Li Y, Tung R, Parker L, Piliang MP, Zins JE. Complications following injection of soft-tissue fillers. Aesthet Surg J. 2013;33(6):862–77.
4. Sykes JM. Commentary on: new high dose pulsed hyaluronidase protocol for hyaluronic acid filler vascular adverse events. Aesthet Surg J. 2017;37(7):826–7.
5. Tansatit T, Apinuntrum P, Phetudom T. A dark side of the cannula injections: how arterial wall perforations and emboli occur. Aesthet Plast Surg. 2017;41(1):221–7.

Visual Complications of Filler Injections

6

Blindness is the most tragic complication of filler injections. The pathophysiology of blindness is known, but its prevention and treatment remain to be elucidated. Many studies have examined this problem.

The incidence of filler injection-induced blindness is increasing. We reviewed all reported cases and found 50 up to September 2018. The most common causes of the increasing incidence of blindness are the rapidly increasing number of filler injections and improper injection techniques. Many cases of blindness can be prevented if the operator uses proper injection technique.

Here we will discuss the pathophysiology, causes, symptoms, treatment, and prevention of ocular complications in an effort to eliminate this tragic complication.

6.1 Incidence of Ocular Complications

Studies on ocular complications usually include autologous fat grafts or unlicensed products; thus, we reviewed all ocular complications by fillers published to date and found 50 cases reported up to September 2018. These 50 cases did not include fat grafts, unknown fillers, or unlicensed products. We analyzed the products that are currently being used. The most common site of ocular complications involved injections at the nasal area, followed by the glabellar area. More than 70% of all ocular complications occur in these two regions.

Ninety percent of ocular complications occur after injections are made into the glabella, nose, forehead, and periocular region, areas that are supplied by the ophthalmic artery branches (Fig. 6.1).

This shows that the ophthalmic artery from internal carotid artery is the main pathway to blindness and we should be very careful when injecting filler into territories of the ophthalmic artery branches.

This new report is different from previous literature because the previous literature usually includes cases of fat graft. Fat grafts should be differentiated from filler injections because the fat graft procedure usually injects large amounts of filler and is much more invasive, disturbing more vessels. The incidence of visual complications by filler injection shows that more than 70% are from glabellar and nasal region injections. This shows that the temple area and mental regions are relatively susceptible to visual complications.

Among all cases reported in the literature through September 2018, 44% were in South Korea (Tables 6.1 and 6.2). Even though Korean doctors are performing a lot of filler injection procedure, it is unreasonable that almost half of all visual complications occur in Korea, and it is estimated that other countries do not report such a high incidence of this tragic complication. The interesting thing about this report is that 84% of all reports are from Korea, China, Taiwan, and Japan because of the relatively higher demand for nasal augmentation by filler injections in Asian countries. This shows that nasal augmentation carries a high risk of blindness.

© Springer Nature Singapore Pte Ltd. 2019
I. S. Koh, W. Lee, *Filler Complications*, https://doi.org/10.1007/978-981-13-6639-0_6

6.2   Pathophysiology

The pathophysiology of filler-related visual disturbances is quite simple. Injected filler is at higher pressure than arterial pressure, and when any ophthalmic artery branch becomes occluded, visual complications occur. Fillers are injected against arterial pressure and regurgitate into the skull por-

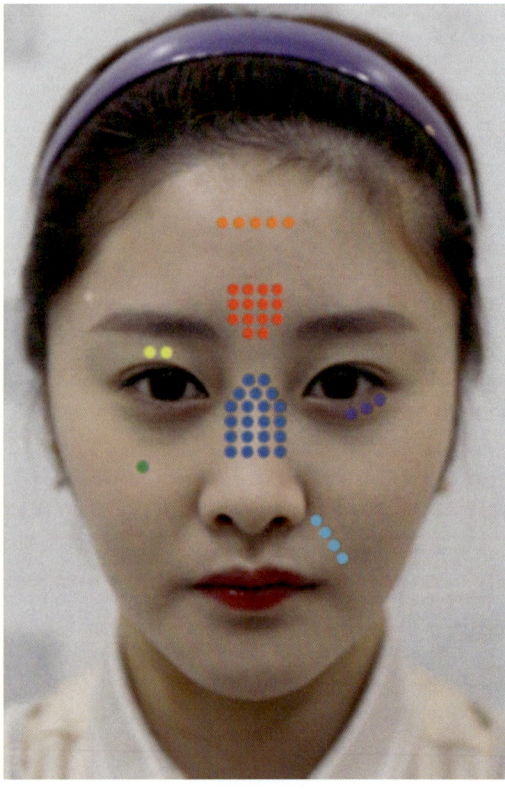

Fig. 6.1 Incidence of ocular complications. We reviewed the literature for articles published through September 2018 and found that the most common site was the nose

Nose	21 (42%)
Glabella	14 (28%)
Forehead	5 (10%)
Periocular	3 (6%)
Upper eyelids	2 (4%)
Nasolabial fold	4 (8%)
Midface	1 (2%)

tion and then run to the ophthalmic artery and occlude nearby branches. Thus, the supratrochlear, supraorbital, and dorsal nasal arteries from internal carotid artery branches and the arteries that connect to the internal carotid artery branches such as the angular and the lateral nasal artery could be the cause of blindness. Inside the skull, the internal carotid artery branches to the ophthalmic, anterior cerebral, middle cerebral, posterior communicating, and anterior choroidal arteries (Fig. 6.2).

The ophthalmic artery is the first branch of the internal carotid artery; when filler regurgitation occurs over this artery, it can cause brain infarction (Fig. 6.3).

The ophthalmic artery is the first branch of the internal carotid artery and anastomoses with the superficial temporal, angular, lateral nasal, and inferior orbital arteries, which arise from the external carotid artery. The most important vessels are the supratrochlear, supraorbital, and dorsal nasal arteries.

The most severe visual disturbance involves occlusion of the central retinal artery. When filler regurgitates proximal to the central retinal artery, the posterior ciliary artery tends to occlude and choroid ischemia occurs (Fig. 6.4).

If the filler is prevented from entering the ophthalmic artery branch, fortunately, it could avoid ocular complications, and skin necrosis might occur.

Blindness involves the following conditions:

1. Filler is injected into an artery that connects to the ophthalmic artery.
2. The entire needle end perforates the arterial lumen.
3. Filler is injected against arterial pressure.
4. Filler amount should be sufficient to fill the arterial lumen located from the entry point to the central retinal artery.

In the first condition of blindness, the filler is injected into an artery that anastomoses to the ophthalmic artery. The ophthalmic artery branches into the supraorbital, supratrochlear, and dorsal nasal

Table 6.1 National incidence of injection filler-induced blindness in the literature

Korea	China	Taiwan	Japan	USA	Canada	Brazil	Germany	Netherlands
22	11	6	3	4	1	1	1	1

Table 6.2 Cases of visual compromise in the literature, September 2018

	Age/sex	Type	Site	Site	Initial symptom	Final symptom	Diagnosis	Systemic	Ocular pain	Ptosis	Ocular motility	Skin necrosis	Country references
1	48/M	HA	Glabella and cheeks	Rt.	Decreased vision Visual field defect	Decreased vision	BRAO	–	–	–	–	–	Germany [2]
2	30/F	HA	Nasal tip and bridge	Lt.	NLP	NLP	CRAO	Headache	+	+	+	+	Korea [3]
3	44/F	HA	Nose	Lt.	Decreased vision	20/1000	AION	Headache	–	–	–	–	China [4]
4	45/F	HA	Periorbital	Rt.	Counting fingers	Counting fingers	CRAO	–	–	–	–	–	China [4]
5	25/F	HA	Forehead	Lt.	Hand movement	2/1000	Incomplete	–	–	–	–	–	China [4]
6	38/F	HA	Upper eyelid	Lt.	NLP	NLP	OAO	Dizziness Vomiting	–	+	+	–	China [4]
7	23/F	HA	Nose	Rt.	NLP	NLP	OAO	Dizziness Vomiting	+	+	+	–	China [4]
8	Young/F	HA	Nasal dorsum	Rt.	NLP	NLP	CRAO	ND	+	+	+	–	Korea [5]
9	Late 30s/M	HA	Forehead	Lt.	20/30	20/25	BRAO	ND	–	–	–	–	US [6]
10	32/F	HA	Nasolabial fold and glabella	Rt.	NLP	NLP	OAO	–	+	+	+	–	Korea [7]
11	26/F	HA	Nasolabial fold	Lt.	Decreased vision Visual field defect	Decreased vision	BRAO	–	–	–	–	–	Korea [7]
12	26/F	HA	Glabella	Lt.	Decreased vision Visual field defect	Decreased vision	BRAO	–	–	–	–	–	Korea [7]
13	26/F	HA	Nasolabial fold	Rt.	Decreased vision Visual field defect	Decreased vision	BRAO	–	–	–	–	–	Korea [7]

(continued)

Table 6.2 (continued)

	Age/sex	Type	Site	Site	Initial symptom	Final symptom	Diagnosis	Systemic	Ocular pain	Ptosis	Ocular motility	Skin necrosis	Country references
14	20/F	HA	Nose	Rt.	Decreased vision	0.6	BRAO	Headache Nausea	+	+	+	+	Korea [8]
15	23/M	HA	Nose	Rt.	NLP	NLP	CRAO	Limb paralysis Dizziness	+	+	+	+	Korea [9]
16	52/M	HA	Nose	R/L	NLP	NLP	CRAO	Headache Brain infarction	+	−	−	+	Taiwan [10]
17	25/F	HA	Glabella	Lt.	NLP	NLP	G PCAO	−	+	+	+	−	Korea [1]
18	39/F	HA	Glabella	Rt.	NLP	NLP	CRAO	−	−	−	−	−	Korea [1]
19	30/M	HA	Nasolabial fold	Rt.	Hand motion	20/25	L PCAO	−	+	+	+	−	Korea [1]
20	22/F	HA	Glabella	Lt.	Decreased vision 20/32	20/25	L PCAO	−	−	+	+	−	Korea [1]
21	46/F	HA	Glabella	Rt.	Decreased vision 20/200	20/63	BRAO	−	−	+	+	−	Korea [1]
22	42/F	HA	Glabella	Rt.	Decreased vision 20/500	20/100	BRAO	−	−	+	+	−	Korea [1]
23	27/F	HA	Glabella and nasal dorsum	Rt.	Light perception	Light perception	PION	−	+	+	+	−	Korea [1]
24	23/F	HA	Nose	Lt.	NLP	NLP	BRAO PION	−	−	+	−	−	China [11]
25	23/F	HA	Nose	Rt.	Hand motion	20/60	BRAO	−	−	+	+	−	China [11]
26	35/F	HA	Nose	Lt.	NLP	NLP	OAO	−	−	+	−	−	China [11]
27	28/F	HA	Forehead	Lt.	20/200	NLP	PION	−	−	+	+	−	China [11]
28	39/F	HA	Midface	Rt.	Blurred vision	Restored Hyaluronidase	ND	Headache Dizziness	+	−	−	−	US [12]
29	20/F	HA	Glabella	Rt.	NLP	NLP	OAO	Nausea	+	−	−	−	Japan [13]
30	41/F	HA	Forehead	Rt.	NLP	Hand motion	PCAO	Limb weakness	+	+	+	+	China [14]
31	50/F	HA	Glabella	Lt.	Hand motion	NLP	CRAO	Brain infarction	−	+	+	−	Korea [15]
32	29/F	HA	Nasal tip	Rt.	Blurred vision	20/20	Oculomotor nerve	Dizziness	+	+	+	+	Korea [16]

No.	Age/Sex	Filler	Location	Side	Vision	Vision	Complication	Systemic symptoms					Country
33	23/F	HA	Nasal dorsum	Rt.	NLP	NLP	CRAO	–	–	–	+	+	US [17]
34	26/F	HA	Nasal dorsum	R/L	NLP	NLP	OAO	–	–	–	–	–	Netherland [18]
35	25/F	HA	Nasal dorsum	Lt.	Blurred vision	20/20	BRAO	–	+	+	+	+	Korea [19]
36	25/F	HA	Nasal dorsum	Rt.	NLP	NLP	BRAO	–	+	+	+	+	China [20]
37	25/F	HA	Nasal dorsum	Rt.	NLP	NLP	CRAO	Brain infarction	+	+	+	–	Taiwan [21]
38	30/M	CaHA	Nasal dorsum	R/L	NLP	NLP	CRAO	–	–	+	+	+	Korea [22]
39	25/M	CaHA	Nasal dorsum	Rt.	Hand motion	20/40	AION	–	+	+	+	+	Korea [23]
40	32/F	CaHA	Glabella	R/L	NLP	Hand motion	BRAO	–	–	–	–	–	Taiwan [24]
41	35/F	CaHA	Nasal dorsum	Lt.	Blurred vision	Hand motion	Choroid	Headache Nausea	+	+	+	+	Taiwan [25]
42	26/F	CaHA	Glabella	Lt.	Blurred vision	20/20	Choroid	Unconsciousness	–	–	+	+	Japan [26]
43	24/F	CaHA	Nasal dorsum	Lt.	Blurred vision	20/20	Choroid	Headache Vomiting	+	+	+	+	Taiwan [27]
44	43/F	PLLA	Periorbital and lateral nasal	Lt.	Vision loss	Light perception	BRAO	Nausea	+	+	+	–	Canada [28]
45	46/F	PLLA	Eyelid	Rt.	NLP	NLP	G PCAO	–	+	+	+	–	Korea [5]
46	55/F	PLLA	Glabella	Lt.	Hand motion	Hand motion	L PCAO	–	–	–	–	–	Korea [5]
47	57/F	PAAG	Periocular	Lt.	Visual field defect 20/70	Visual field defect 20/30	AION	Headache Nausea	–	–	+	+	Taiwan [29]
48	Mid 40/F	PMMA	Forehead	Rt.	NLP	Faint light perception	BRAO	–	–	–	–	–	US [6]
49	52/F	PMMA	Glabella	Rt.	NLP	NLP	ND	–	+	–	+	–	Brazil [30]
50	29/M	PMMA	Nasal dorsum	Rt.	NLP	NLP	CRAO	–	+	+	+	–	Japan [31]

HA Hyaluronic acid, *CaHA* Calcium hydroxyapatite, *PMMA* Polymethyl methacrylate, *PLLA* Poly-L-lactic acid, *PAAG* Polyacrylamide, *ND* Not described, *NLP* No light perception, *OAO* Ophthalmic artery occlusion, *CRAO* Central retinal artery occlusion, *PCAO* Posterior ciliary artery occlusion, *AION* Anterior ischemic optic neuropathy, *PION* Posterior ischemic optic neuropathy, *BRAO* Branch of retinal artery occlusion

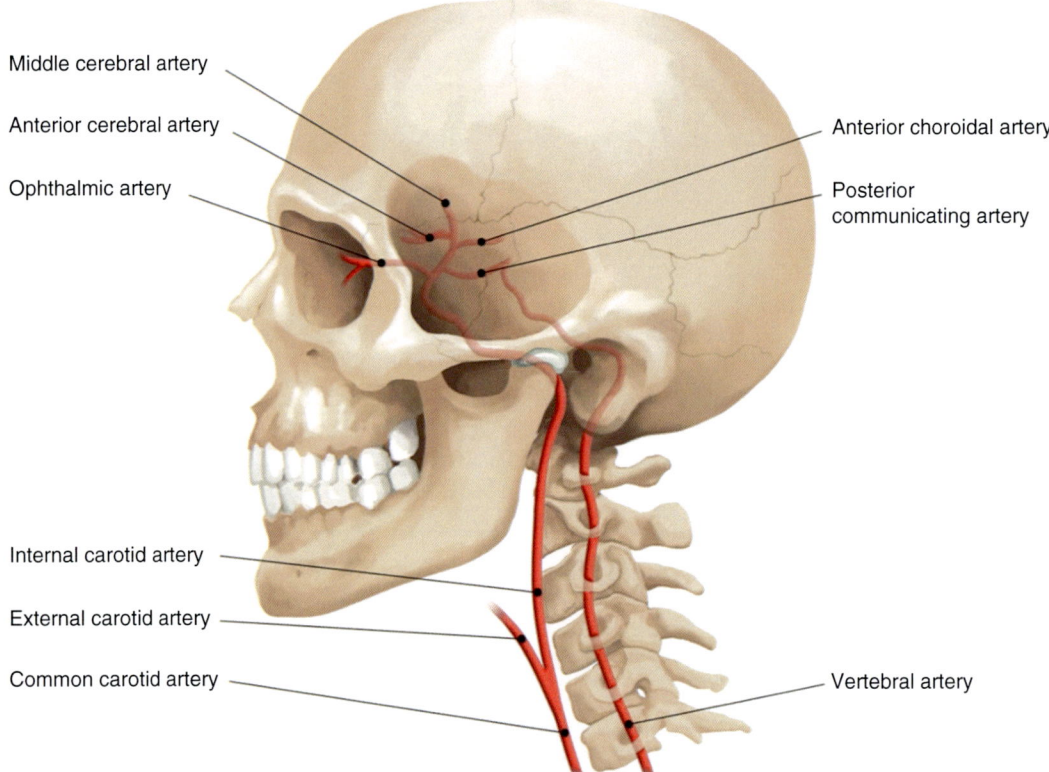

Fig. 6.2 Internal carotid artery pathway

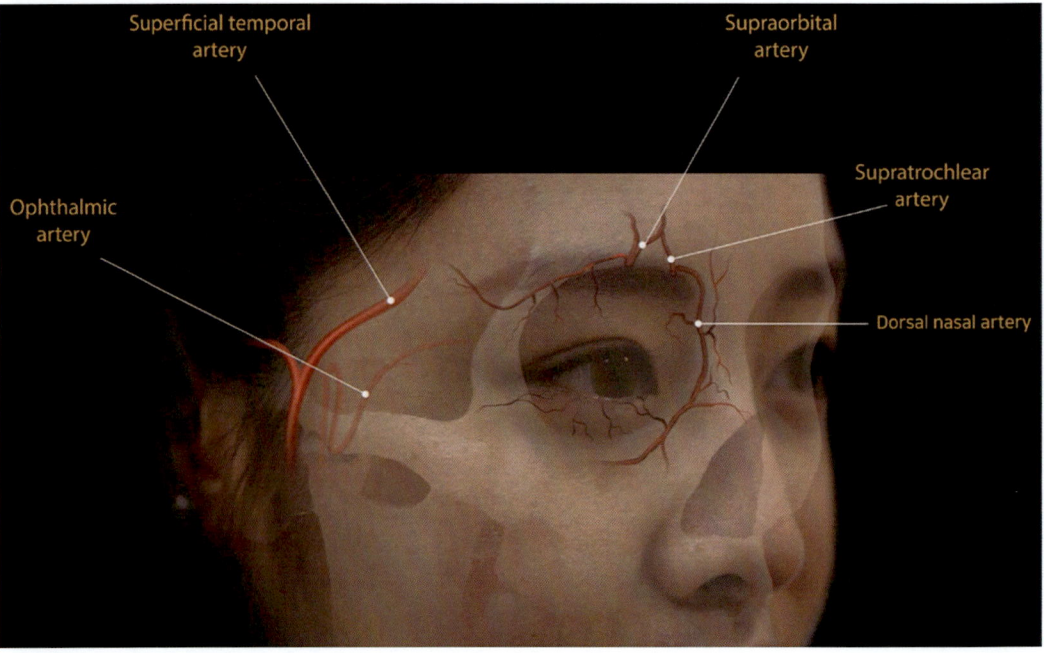

Fig. 6.3 Ophthalmic artery anastomosis arteries. The ophthalmic artery branches from the internal carotid artery to the supratrochlear, supraorbital, and dorsal nasal arteries

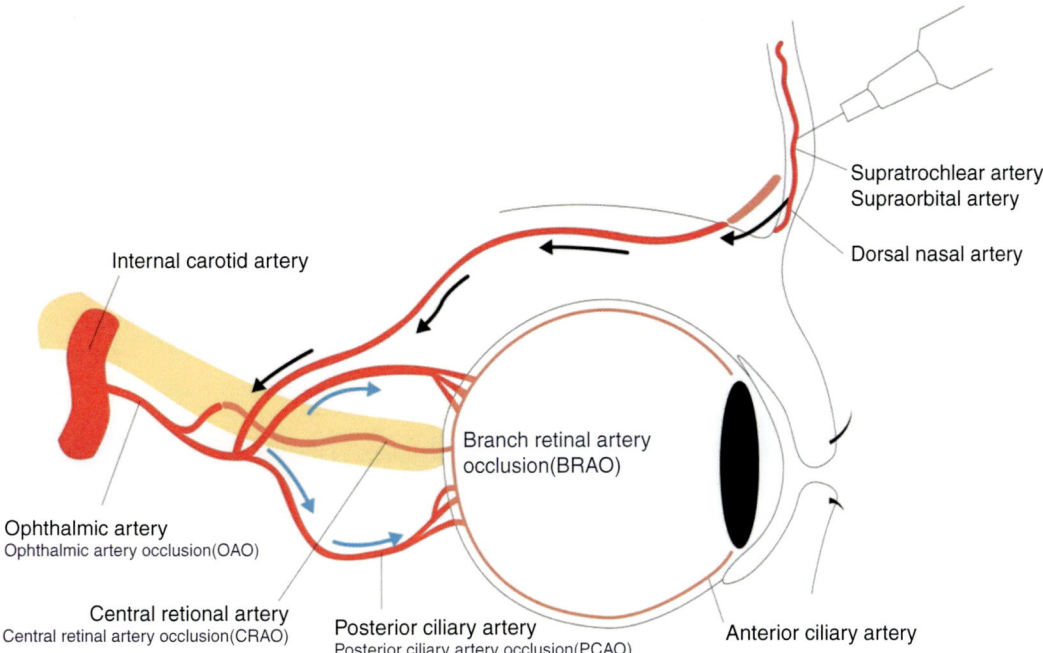

Fig. 6.4 Pathophysiology of blindness. Filler injection into the supratrochlear, supraorbital, or dorsal nasal artery causes ocular complications via regurgitation into the ophthalmic artery, and the location of the embolism indicates the extent of complications

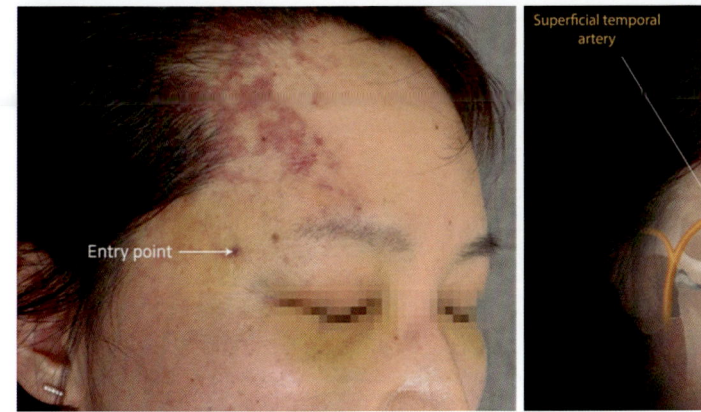

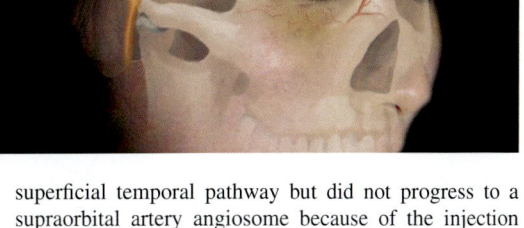

Fig. 6.5 Distal extended necrosis after filler injection into the superficial temporal artery. Skin necrosis occurred 4 days after the injection of 1.5 mL hyaluronic acid filler into the temple area. Skin necrosis developed along the superficial temporal pathway but did not progress to a supraorbital artery angiosome because of the injection being made in the opposite direction

arteries, in which regurgitation can easily occur that reaches the central retinal artery because they are directly connected to each other. On the other hand, arteries arising from the external carotid artery such as superficial temporal and lateral nasal arteries are also connected to the ophthalmic artery but have their own pathway, making regurgitation into the ophthalmic artery anastomosis less likely. Previous studies described blindness cases after injections into the temple area, but since we excluded fat graft cases, we encountered no cases of injection-induced blindness (Figs. 6.1 and 6.5).

Blindness caused by a nasolabial fold injection occurred in 8% (4/50) cases in our study (Fig. 6.1). The angular and lateral nasal arteries are branches of the facial artery that arise from the external carotid artery. These two vessels are connected to the dorsal nasal artery by the internal carotid artery branch. When filler is injected into the angular and lateral nasal arteries, it tends to run in the forward direction; when it reaches the dorsal nasal artery, it should run in the opposite direction. This is the same mechanism by which the superficial temporal artery connects to the supraorbital artery; it should run in the opposite direction against arterial pressure to cause blindness (Fig. 6.6).

Filler injected at the nasolabial fold runs in the forward direction at the angular artery and the lateral nasal artery; however, when it reaches the dorsal nasal artery, the flow should regurgitate against the pressure to enter to ophthalmic artery. However, we hypothesize that ocular complications in cases of nasolabial fold injection can occur for reasons including the following:

1. A large amount of filler is injected into the nasolabial fold that then enters the artery.
2. Nasolabial fold correction is performed much more commonly than temple augmentation.
3. Dorsal nasal arterial pressure is relatively low and regurgitation occurs easily.

Cases such as that shown in Fig. 6.7 are commonly encountered. Even when the filler is not injected directly into the dorsal nasal artery, injections into connected arteries such as the lateral nasal or angular arteries can easily cause regurgitation into the dorsal nasal artery. Thus,

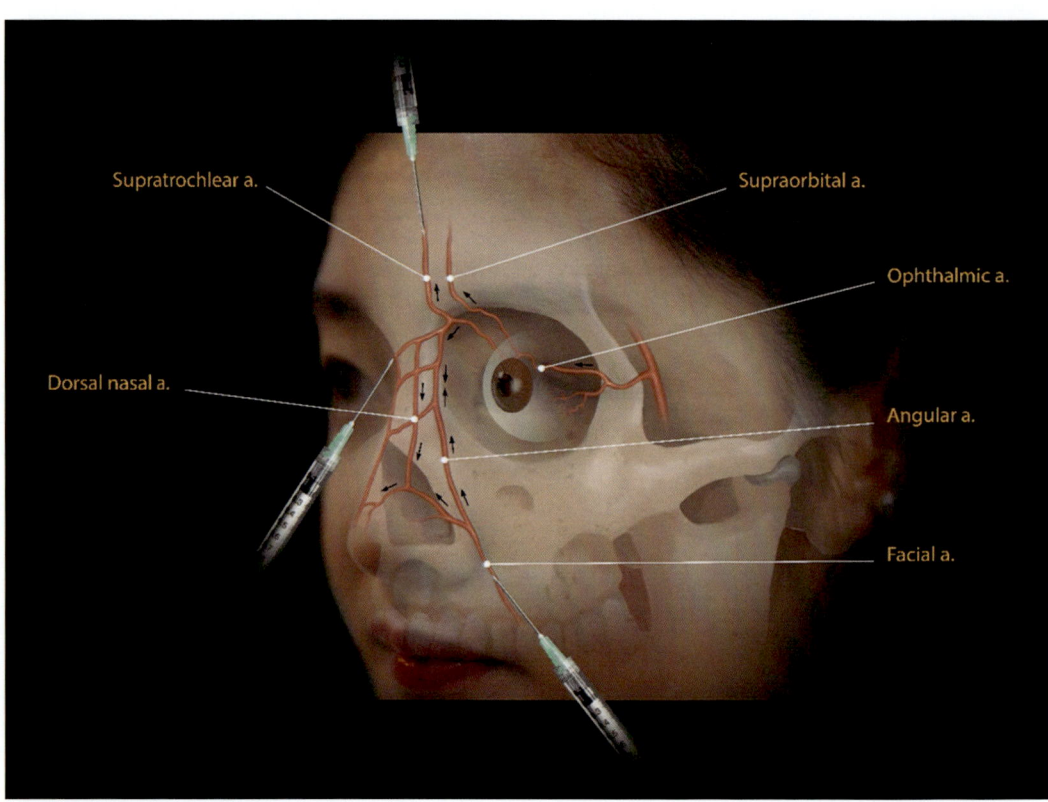

Fig. 6.6 Pathophysiology of ocular complications of injecting at the nasolabial fold. The facial artery located at the nasolabial fold area arises from the external carotid artery branch and is relatively safe from the internal carotid artery branches. However, the facial artery is connected to the dorsal nasal artery, and high-pressure injections here might induce ocular complications

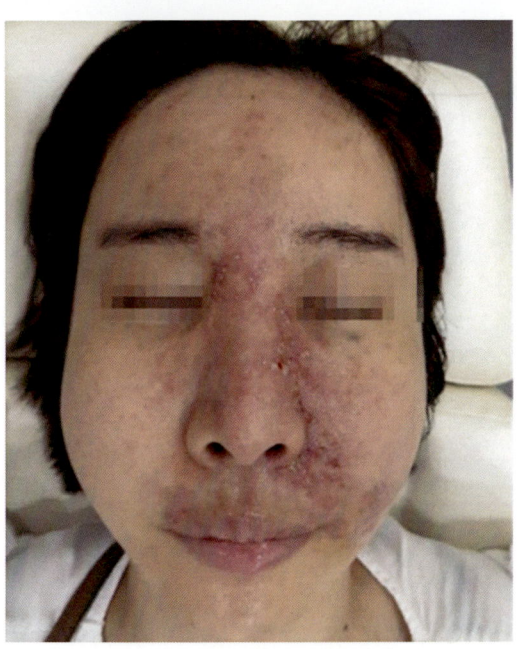

Table 6.3 Needle diameters

	Outer diameter (mm)	Inner diameter (mm)
18G	1.27	0.84
19.5G	0.99	0.69
21G	0.82	0.51
22G	0.71	0.41
23G	0.64	0.34
25G	0.51	0.26
27G	0.41	0.21
29G	0.34	0.18
30G	0.31	0.16

Fig. 6.7 Three days after the hyaluronic acid filler is injected into the nasolabial fold. Filler was injected into the left nasolabial fold and skin necrosis developed because the filler moved in the forward direction through the dorsal nasal artery territory and created a contralateral supratrochlear artery angiosome

when injections are made into the nasolabial fold, caution should be taken to prevent entry into the dorsal nasal artery pathway.

The second condition of ocular complications is that the entire needle should fit within the arterial lumen. The important thing about this condition is that the injection pressure is transferred into the vessel and filler can migrate to areas with higher pressure. The use of a larger-diameter needle carries a higher risk of vessel injury but a decreased risk of the needle puncturing the vessel. Thus, in cases in which a vessel is punctured by a large-diameter needle, the pressure is distributed and cannot reach distant locations. A review of the literature revealed that the supratrochlear, supraorbital, and dorsal nasal arteries have approximately 1 mm diameters. A relatively large-diameter needle (23G) has a small outer diameter (0.64 mm) that can be inserted into a 1-mm-diameter artery. Many doctors like to use 27G needles, which have an outer diameter of

0.41 mm and can be easily be inserted into an artery (Table 6.3, Fig. 6.8).

The third condition of visual complications is that there should be enough injection pressure to overcome arterial pressure and frictional force of the vessel wall. To reach the central retinal artery, regurgitation into the ophthalmic artery is necessary, which requires a high-pressure injection. Clinically, a needle with a smaller diameter is required to create a high-pressure injection. High pressure is needed when injecting using a small-diameter needle than a large-diameter needle. Also, when a biphasic filler is injected, a small-diameter needle could become occluded by large particles, so relatively higher pressure is needed. If occlusion is felt during the filler injection procedure, it is better to stop the injection and possibly change the needle.

The fourth condition is that a large amount of filler is needed to occlude a vessel from the entry point to the central retinal artery. Thus, when the entry point is far from the eye, there is a lower chance of blindness. It is also true that a small amount of filler could result in complications when injections are made at the nose, glabella, or periorbital area because the distance is short.

Regarding these conditions, the most important locations are the internal carotid artery branches, i.e., the supratrochlear, supraorbital, and dorsal nasal arteries are the most dangerous locations (Fig. 6.9). Thus, clinicians should always monitor for the risk of blindness when performing filler injections to the nose, forehead, glabella, and periorbital areas.

Fig. 6.8 Arterial diameter compared to cannula diameter. The diameters of the supratrochlear, supraorbital, and dorsal nasal arteries are approximately 1 mm

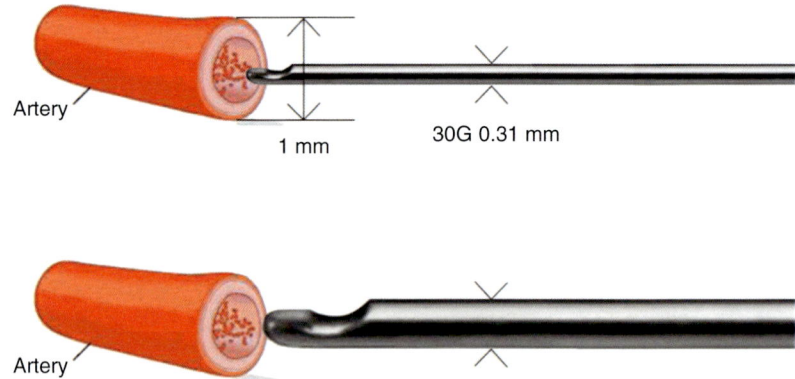

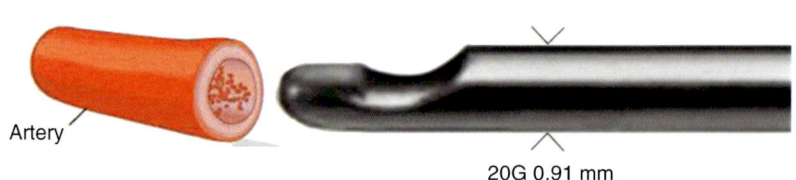

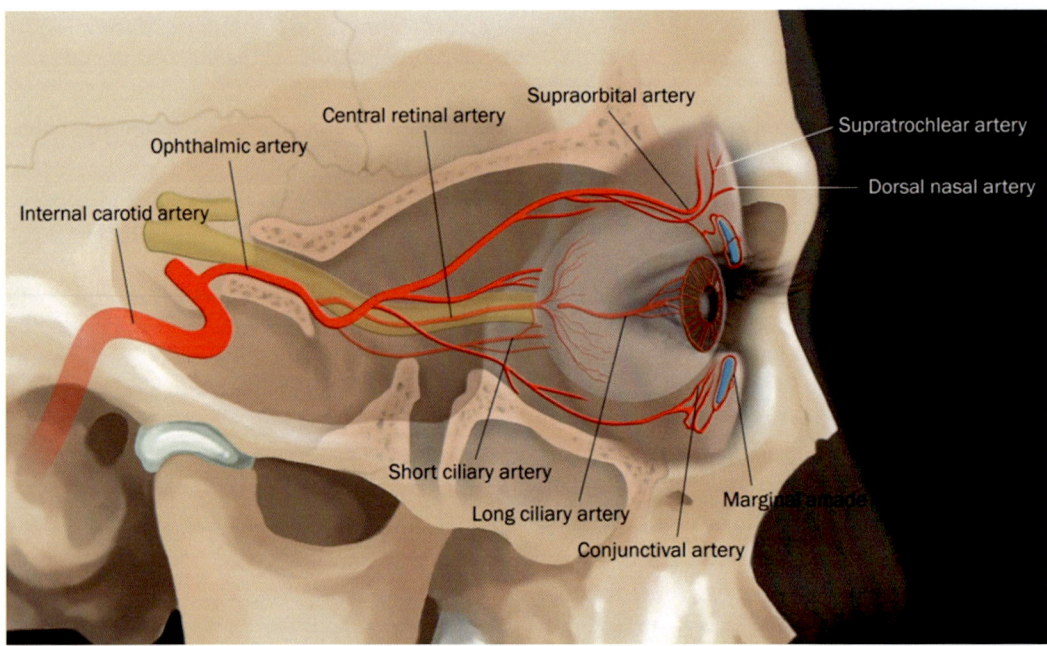

Fig. 6.9 Ophthalmic artery pathway. The supratrochlear, supraorbital, and dorsal nasal arteries arise from the ophthalmic artery branches. One should also work with care in the periorbital area

6.3 Symptoms

Sudden severe pain is the most common symptom of blindness. Blurred vision, hemianopsia, decreased visual acuity, skin necrosis, and blepharoptosis could also occur. The symptoms are related to the arteries that are occluded by the regurgitation. When filler is injected into the supratrochlear, supraorbital, and dorsal nasal arteries and cannot reach the ophthalmic artery, only skin necrosis would occur. However, when more filler is regurgitated into the ophthalmic artery, PION, BRAO, CRAO, LPCAO, GPCAO, and OAO might occur. Even when regurgitation into the internal carotid artery occurs, a brain infarction also might occur. Thus, the symptoms and skin necrosis patterns can indicate which artery has been affected (Fig. 6.10).

Recovering from blindness is very difficult; in some recovery cases, the first symptom is partial visual loss. Thus, the prognosis is very much related with the first symptoms.

The most important thing might be when said symptoms occur. Many studies have suggested multiple treatments, but the pupillary light reflex must be checked first (Fig. 6.11). This examina-

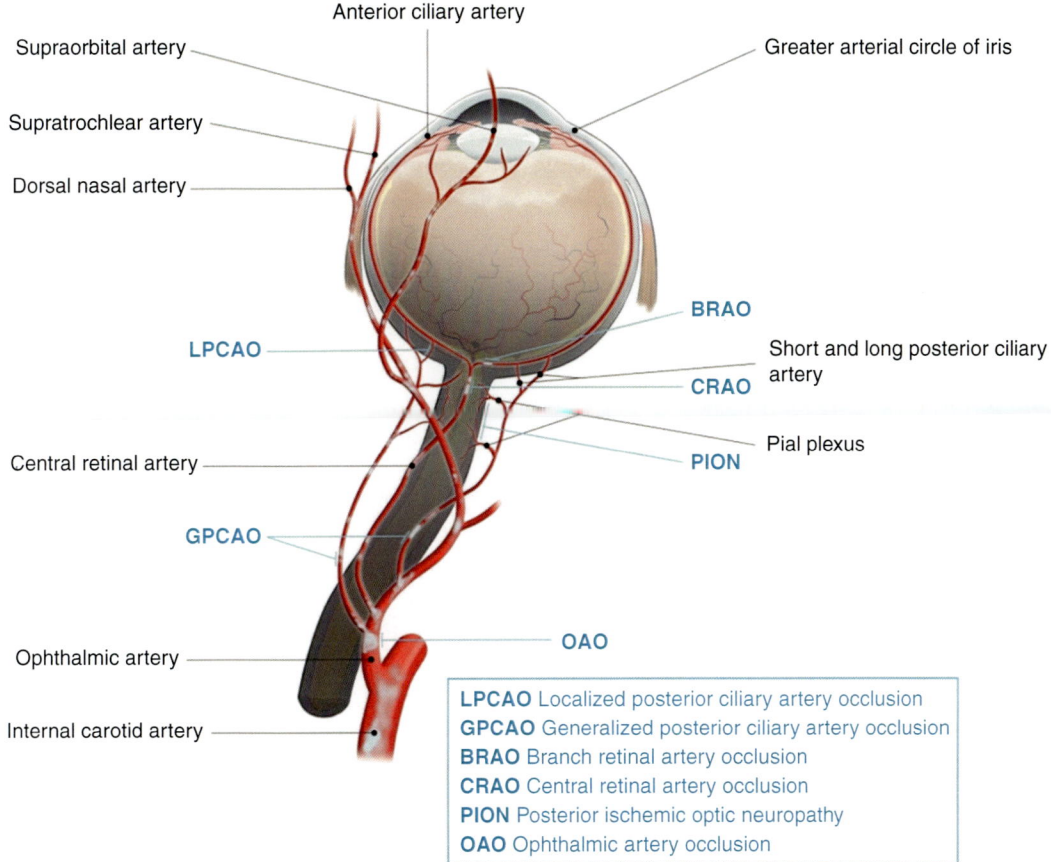

Supraorbital artery

Anterior ciliary artery

Supratrochlear artery

Dorsal nasal artery

Greater arterial circle of iris

BRAO

LPCAO

Short and long posterior ciliary artery

CRAO

Central retinal artery

Pial plexus

PION

GPCAO

OAO

Ophthalmic artery

Internal carotid artery

LPCAO Localized posterior ciliary artery occlusion
GPCAO Generalized posterior ciliary artery occlusion
BRAO Branch retinal artery occlusion
CRAO Central retinal artery occlusion
PION Posterior ischemic optic neuropathy
OAO Ophthalmic artery occlusion

Fig. 6.10 Symptoms and diagnosis of ocular complications. When filler is injected into the internal carotid artery, brain infarction might occur, leading to severe acute pain in the ophthalmic artery and even blindness. A visual disturbance that occurs a few minutes after the filler injection such as a branched retinal artery occlusion might recover spontaneously

Fig. 6.11 Pupillary light reflex. When there is an ocular symptom after the filler injection, the first examination should include checking the direct and indirect light reflexes. When there is no pupillary constriction, treatment such as a retrobulbar hyaluronidase injection should be considered before the transfer

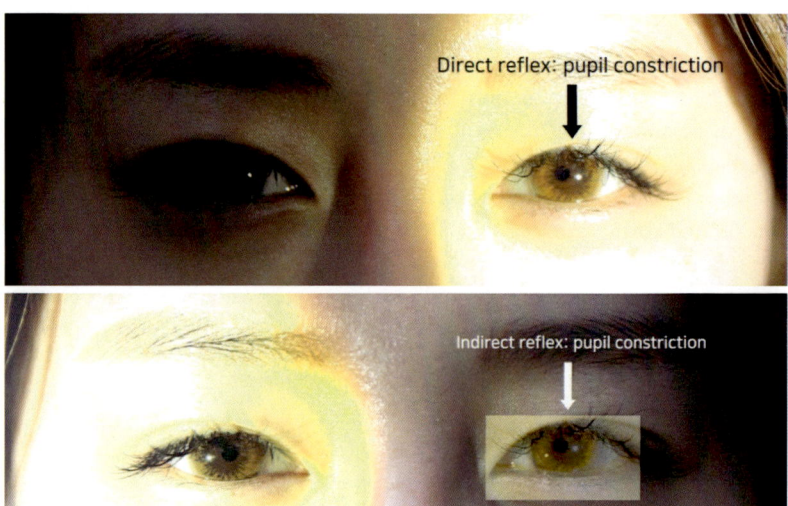

tion is not diagnostic; rather, it is the only tool that can screen for real ocular problems. If pupillary dilatation is present, one should consider using a retrobulbar hyaluronidase injection instead.

6.4   Treatments

6.4.1   Emergency Treatment

There is no definite treatment for ocular complications. Many studies have described many treatments, but none are evidence-based. However, the following treatment guidelines should be considered.

> **Emergency Treatment**
> 1. Call 911.
> 2. Check direct and indirect light reflexes.
> 3. Timolol 0.5% 1–2 drops per eye
> 4. Consider retrobulbar hyaluronidase injection.
> 5. Ocular massage: press eyeball 10–15 seconds and suddenly release the pressure. Repeat for 3–5 minutes.
> 6. Treatment after transfer:
>   IV acetazolamide 500 mg
>   IV mannitol
>   IV heparin
>   Hyperbaric oxygen therapy
>   IV corticosteroids

The purpose of ocular massage is to recanalize vessel by pressure differences. Timolol reduces ocular pressure, while acetazolamide decreases ocular pressures and increases retinal perfusion.

6.4.2   Retrobulbar Hyaluronidase Injection

The retrobulbar injection of hyaluronidase is the first treatment that should be considered in cases of blindness symptoms. Although its effectiveness remains to be confirmed, one study reported on its use to cure blindness. Not all doctors are familiar with this technique, but if this method can cure the complications, it should be performed. It is advisable that clinicians prepare for this tragic complication because the injection should be performed as soon as possible.

Technique: The distance between the anterior orbital margin and the retrobulbar space is at least 25 mm, so a long (38 mm) needle should be used. The needle length is generally 18G. The use of a 25G long needle or long cannula is also acceptable (Fig. 6.12). The entry point should be the lateral part of the orbital rim and the orbital bone scratched by the needle tip to approach the retrobulbar space. This is not a difficult procedure. We strongly suggest that clinicians practice the retrobulbar injection technique in a cadaver dissection workshop.

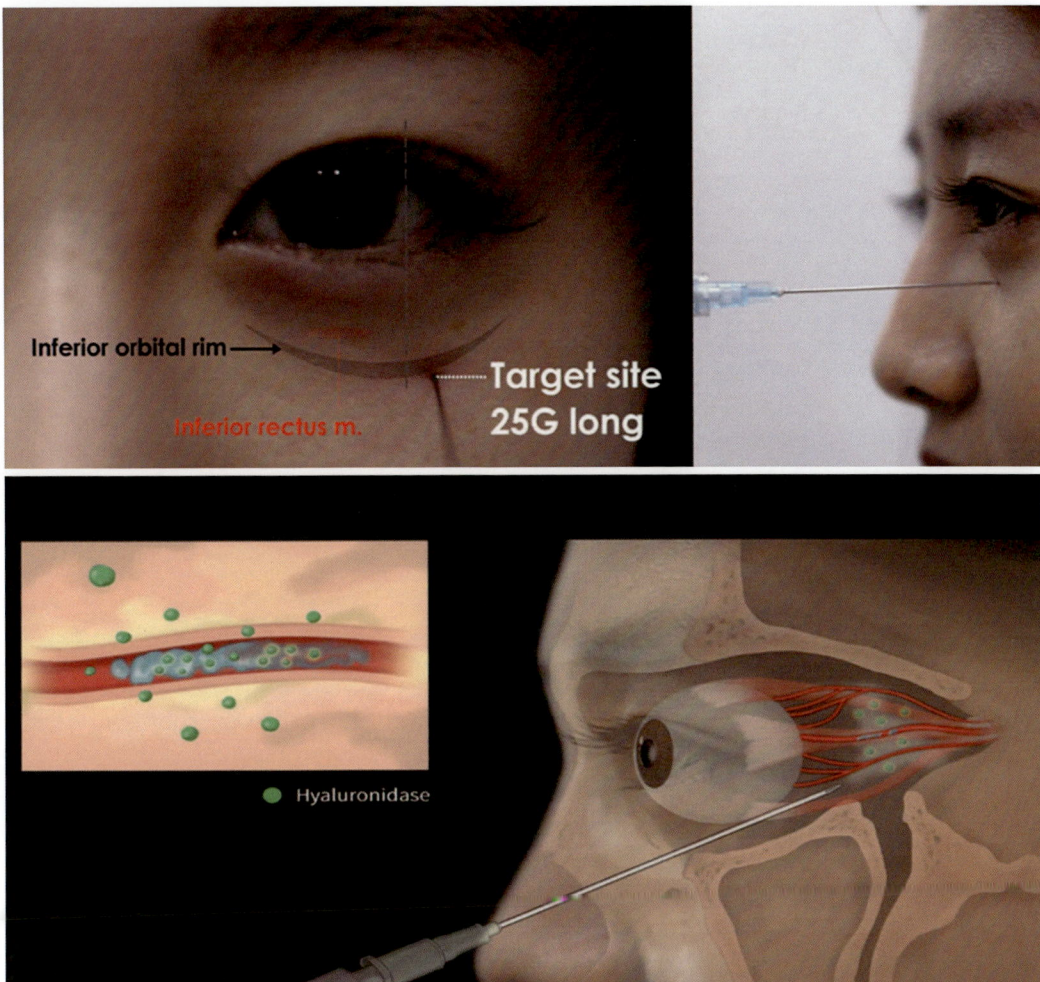

Fig. 6.12 Retrobulbar hyaluronidase injection technique. First, draw a virtual vertical line from the lateral canthal line and approach at inferior orbital rim with the needle or cannula. Next, scratch the orbital floor and feel orbital bone and approach at least 2.5 cm posteriorly, and inject into the retrobulbar space. Hyaluronidase separates into hyaluronic acid by diffusion, so it is important to make the injection as soon as possible

The proper dosage of the retrobulbar hyaluronidase injection has yet to be determined, but we recommend the injection of 1500 IU first, followed by 1500 IU. Previous studies described the injection of 400–800 USP, but since the United States markets 200 USP per bottle, the amount would be not enough. Since this is a tragic complication, authors like to recommend to inject as much as possible.

One author recently induced iatrogenic blindness by filler injections in rabbits and found that the retrobulbar injection of 3000 IU of hyaluronidase reversed the condition.

6.4.3 Emergency Kit

It is very important to have an emergency kit available because doctors tend to panic when filler complications such as skin necrosis and ocular complications occur (Fig. 6.13).

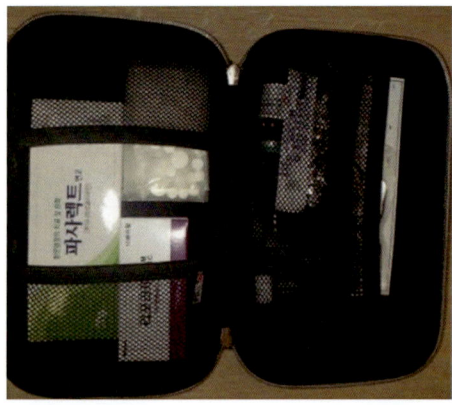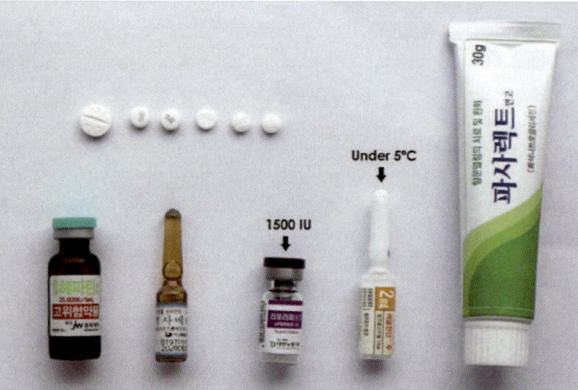

Fig. 6.13 Emergency kit for filler complications

There are emergency drugs for blindness and skin necrosis. It is advisable not to use nitroglycerin paste because of the risk of vessel choking, so a doctor should prepare their own medical knowledge.

Author's Emergency Kit
1. Hyaluronidase 1500 IU
2. Timolol 0.25% eye drops
3. Nitroglycerine paste
4. IV – Prostaglandin E1 2 mL stored at <5 °C
    Dexamethasone
    Heparin 5000 U
5. Po: Opalmon
    Ciprobay 260 mg
    Methylprednisolone 4 mg
    Aspirin 100 mg

6.5   Prevention

Prevention in such a tragic complication is critical. To achieve proper prevention, proper techniques must be used. Here are some suggestions.

6.5.1   Anatomy

The most important prevention is knowledge of the anatomy. Specifically, knowledge of the loca-tions of the supratrochlear, supraorbital, and dorsal nasal arteries is extremely important.

6.5.2   Aspiration

Aspiration before a filler injection remains controversial. It is quite important when a needle tip punctures a large-diameter vessel, as small-diameter vessels tend to shrink during aspiration, whereas large-diameter vessels do not. Also, when a needle is filled with filler, it is difficult to aspirate blood. Many studies have described that aspiration could not be performed by a small-diameter needle. Another point is that the needle tip moves during the injection, so complete prevention is impossible. However, for large-diameter vessels such as the supra-trochlear, supraorbital, and dorsal nasal arteries, aspiration should be checked before the filler injections.

6.5.3   Big Cannula/Needle

Using a large versus small needle is controver-sial, but we strongly advise using a relatively large-diameter cannula or needle (>23G). A larger-diameter needle needs a relatively low injection force. Actually, high pressure is one of the more common reasons for skin necrosis or blindness, so it is very important to control the pressure. Also, a smaller-diameter needle can more easily enter a vessel than a larger-diameter needle, creating an embolism. Finally, a large-diameter needle can be used to perform aspiration prior to the filler injection, so the use of a 23G or larger cannula or needle is highly recommended.

6.5.4 Compression

The easiest preventive method is compression of the arterial pathway. When the injection is made into the dorsum of the nose, bilateral compression should be applied at the dorsal nasal arteries. When injecting into the glabella, one should compress the supratrochlear pathway; when injecting into the forehead, one should compress the supratrochlear notch and supraorbital notch area. These two vessels are anastomosed to each other, so blocking both pathways is important (Figs. 6.14 and 6.15).

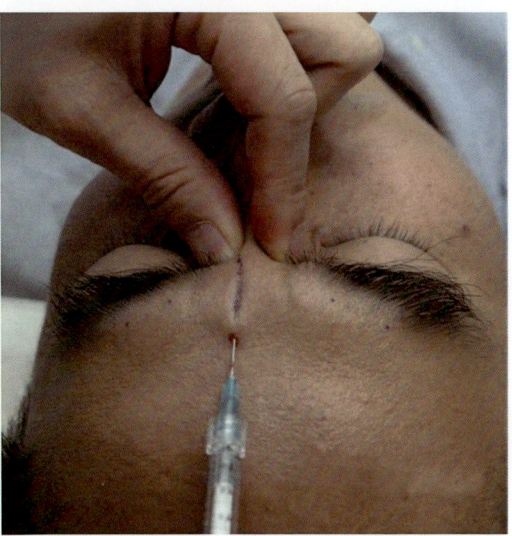

Fig. 6.15 Supratrochlear artery compression. A compression technique is used to prevent regurgitation of the supratrochlear artery when correcting the glabella

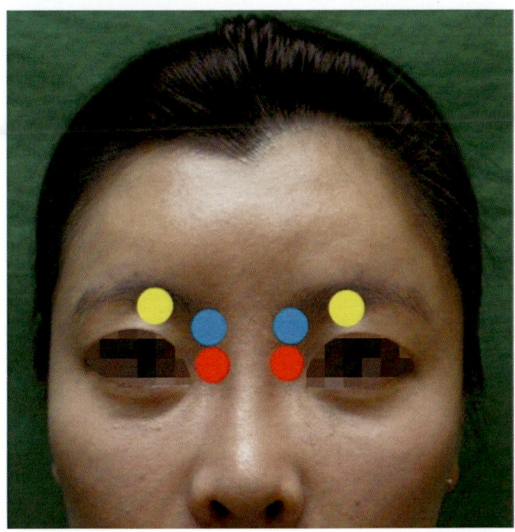

Fig. 6.14 Compression location. Red: Dorsal nasal artery pathway after injection into the dorsum of the nose. Blue: Supratrochlear artery pathway after injection into the glabella. Yellow: Supraorbital artery pathway after injection into the forehead. It is advisable to compress the supratrochlear artery pathway concomitantly

6.5.5 Direction

Injection direction should be parallel to the artery and from the proximal to the distal direction. When the direction of injection is perpendicular to the artery, the probability of puncture is increased. And arteries tend to be shallow when they run distally, so less chance of puncture at distal location.

Thus, this rule should be followed, but in some places like glabella injections, it should be performed in opposite direction and more care should be taken.

6.5.6 Epinephrine

Epinephrine causes vasoconstriction, so it might be useful to avoid vascular compromise. But also it could not differentiate from the first sign of filler-induced vascular occlusion which is pale skin change. Using epinephrine with lidocaine has advantages such as less pain, less bleeding, and less swelling.

6.5.7   Filler Injection Technique

Single bolus injection and linear threading technique have their own advantages and disadvantages. Linear threading technique cannot avoid vessel when the first passage tears the vessel. Thus, the single bolus technique is preferred. While performing the single bolus technique, vessel trauma should always be assessed first, and then a large volume should be injected at one location. In this method, there should be a 5 seconds gap between the puncture and injection to check for bleeding. When there is no bleeding, it is quite safe to inject. Most importantly, the avascular plane should be injected.

6.5.8   Gentle Injection

To inject with minimal pressure is absolutely important. To reduce pressure, injection should be performed using a big diameter needle and small volume syringe. Using a small diameter needle can help to improve the precision of injection, but it has a risk of vascular compromise. Gentle and smooth injection is absolutely important.

6.5.9   History

Previous operation history should be checked because normal vasculature has been changed during operation. For example, forehead augmentation with implant or rhinoplasty with implant would distort normal vasculature because of the implant and the capsule surrounding the implants. Also, previous operative lesions are not flexible, and the filler injected with more pressure increases the chance of vascular compromise.

In particular, previous open rhinoplasty patients with damaged columellar arteries should be careful of filler injections.

6.5.10   Injection by Cannula or Needle

The choice of needle or cannula is always controversial but should be chosen by considering advantages and disadvantages. Big diameter needle (23G) is preferred, but a lot of doctors like to use small diameter cannula. Advantages and disadvantages are as follows:

Big diameter needles facilitate puncture of the precise layer. When the injector knows anatomical layers, it is definitely easy to use a big diameter to locate precise layer. But the needle tends to damage vessels, and when the tip is moved like cannula, more vessel trauma and more bruising can occur. Blunt microcannula has less chance of vessel trauma, but since the tip is blunt, it is difficult to locate the tip at a definite anatomical layer.

One of the reasons of ocular complications of rhinoplasty is the use of a blunt cannula at infralobular entry point. Long and flexible blunt microcannula tip could locate subcutaneous layer instead of supraperiosteal layer. And this might cause embolism in the dorsal nasal artery and cause blindness (Fig. 6.16).

Therefore, 21G needle is preferred for nose augmentation. 21G is not flexible and has a big

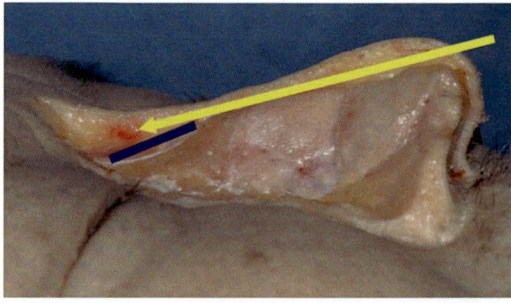

Fig. 6.16 Dangerous technique when using long microcannula at nose augmentation. When using a long cannula or needle, nasal bone angle should be considered (blue line). When the tip is passed through the bony cartilaginous portion, the tip could be located at the subcutaneous layer

diameter and can be used to arrive at the exact layer. However, many doctors fear using this needle and use cannula and should be cautioned. Blunt microcannula can be flexible and locate subcutaneous layer, thus causing dorsal nasal artery trauma.

Preventive Guidelines (ABC Technique)

A. Anatomy: Always avoid subcutaneous layer.

B. Big needle: Bigger than 23G needle or cannula is recommended.

C. Compression: When inject territories of supratrochlear artery, supraorbital artery, dorsal nasal artery, Should compress vessel pathway during injection

D. Direction: Needle should be inserted parallel to arterial pathway.

E. Epinephrine: Minimal use of epinephrine is considerable.

F. Filler injection technique: Single bolus injection is a useful technique.

G. Gentle: Gentle injection with low pressure is extremely important.

H. History: Always check operation history.

Blindness is the most tragic complication and has no definite treatment until today. Therefore, preventive measures need to be elucidated to minimize this complication.

References

1. Park KH, Kim YK, Woo SJ, et al. Iatrogenic occlusion of the ophthalmic artery after cosmetic facial filler injections: a national survey by the Korean Retina Society. JAMA Ophthalmol. 2014;132(6):714–23.
2. Peter S, Mennel S. Retinal branch artery occlusion following injection of hyaluronic acid (Restylane). Clin Exp Ophthalmol. 2006;34(4):363–4.
3. Kim YJ, Kim SS, Song WK, Lee SY, Yoon JS. Ocular ischemia with hypotony after injection of hyaluronic acid gel. Ophthalmic Plast Reconstr Surg. 2011;27(6):e152–5.
4. Chen Y, Wang W, Li J, Yu Y, Li L, Lu N. Fundus artery occlusion caused by cosmetic facial injections. Chin Med J. 2014;127(8):1434–7.
5. Kim SN, Byun DS, Park JH, et al. Panophthalmoplegia and vision loss after cosmetic nasal dorsum injection. J Clin Neurosci. 2014;21(4):678–80.
6. Carle MV, Roe R, Novack R, Boyer DS. Cosmetic facial fillers and severe vision loss. JAMA Ophthalmol. 2014;132(5):637–9.
7. Park SW, Woo SJ, Park KH, Huh JW, Jung C, Kwon OK. Iatrogenic retinal artery occlusion caused by cosmetic facial filler injections. Am J Ophthalmol. 2012;154(4):653–662.e1.
8. Kwon SG, Hong JW, Roh TS, Kim YS, Rah DK, Kim SS. Ischemic oculomotor nerve palsy and skin necrosis caused by vascular embolization after hyaluronic acid filler injection: a case report. Ann Plast Surg. 2013;71(4):333–4.
9. Kim EG, Eom TK, Kang SJ. Severe visual loss and cerebral infarction after injection of hyaluronic acid gel. J Craniofac Surg. 2014;25(2):684–6.
10. He MS, Sheu MM, Huang ZL, Tsai CH, Tsai RK. Sudden bilateral vision loss and brain infarction following cosmetic hyaluronic acid injection. JAMA Ophthalmol. 2013;131(9):1234–5.
11. Zhu GZ, Sun ZS, Liao WX, et al. Efficacy of retrobulbar hyaluronidase injection for vision loss resulting from hyaluronic acid filler embolization. Aesthet Surg J. 2017;38(1):12–22.
12. Chesnut C. Restoration of visual loss with retrobulbar hyaluronidase injection after hyaluronic acid filler. Dermatol Surg. 2018;44(3):435–7.
13. Nonomura S, Oshitari T, Miura G, Chiba A, Yamamoto S. A case of ophthalmic artery occlusion following injection of hyaluronic acid into the glabellar area. Nippon Ganka Gakkai Zasshi. 2014;118(9):783–7.
14. Hu XZ, Hu JY, Wu PS, Yu SB, Kikkawa DO, Lu W. Posterior ciliary artery occlusion caused by hyaluronic acid injections into the forehead: a case report. Medicine (Baltimore). 2016;95(11):e3124.
15. Lee WS, Yoon WT, Choi YJ, Park SP. Multiple cerebral infarctions with neurological symptoms and ophthalmic artery occlusion after filler injection. J Korean Ophthalmol Soc. 2015;56(2):285–90.
16. Bae IH, Kim MS, Choi H, Na CH, Shin BS. Ischemic oculomotor nerve palsy due to hyaluronic acid filler injection. J Cosmet Dermatol. 2018;17:1016.
17. Ramesh S, Fiaschetti D, Goldberg RA. Orbital and ocular ischemic syndrome with blindness after facial

filler injection. Ophthalmic Plast Reconstr Surg. 2018;34:e108–10.

18. Schelke LW, Fick M, van Rijn LJ, Decates T, Velthuis PJ, Niessen F. Unilateral blindness following a non-surgical rhinoplasty with filler. Ned Tijdschr Geneeskd. 2017;161(0):D1246.

19. Lee JI, Kang SJ, Sun H. Skin necrosis with oculomotor nerve palsy due to a hyaluronic acid filler injection. Arch Plast Surg. 2017;44(4):340–3.

20. Chen W, Wu L, Jian XL, et al. Retinal branch artery embolization following hyaluronic acid injection: a case report. Aesthet Surg J. 2016;36(7):NP219–24.

21. Lin YC, Chen WC, Liao WC, Hsia TC. Central retinal artery occlusion and brain infarctions after nasal filler injection. QJM. 2015;108(9):731–2.

22. Kim YJ, Choi KS. Bilateral blindness after filler injection. Plast Reconstr Surg. 2013;131(2):298e–9e.

23. Sung MS, Kim HG, Woo KI, Kim YD. Ocular ischemia and ischemic oculomotor nerve palsy after vascular embolization of injectable calcium hydroxylapatite filler. Ophthalmic Plast Reconstr Surg. 2010;26(4):289–91.

24. Hsiao SF, Huang YH. Partial vision recovery after iatrogenic retinal artery occlusion. BMC Ophthalmol. 2014;14:120.

25. Chou CC, Chen HH, Tsai YY, Li YL, Lin HJ. Choroid vascular occlusion and ischemic optic neuropathy after facial calcium hydroxyapatite injection- a case report. BMC Surg. 2015;15:21.

26. Marumo Y, Hiraoka M, Hashimoto M, Ohguro H. Visual impairment by multiple vascular embolization with hydroxyapatite particles. Orbit. 2018;37(3):165–70.

27. Sung WI, Tsai S, Chen LJ. Ocular complications following cosmetic filler injection. JAMA Ophthalmol. 2018;136(5):e180716.

28. Roberts SA, Arthurs BP. Severe visual loss and orbital infarction following periorbital aesthetic poly-(L)-lactic acid (PLLA) injection. Ophthalmic Plast Reconstr Surg. 2012;28(3):e68–70.

29. Chen YH, Tsai YJ, Chao AN, Huang YS, Kao LY. Visual field defect after facial rejuvenation with botulinum toxin type A and polyacrylamide hydrogel injection. Plast Reconstr Surg. 2010;126(5):249e–50e.

30. Silva MT, Curi AL. Blindness and total ophthalmoplegia after aesthetic polymethylmethacrylate injection: case report. Arq Neuropsiquiatr. 2004;62(3B):873–4.

31. Kubota T, Hirose H. Permanent loss of vision following cosmetic rhinoplastic surgery. Jpn J Ophthalmol. 2005;49(6):535–6.

Index

© Springer Nature Singapore Pte Ltd. 2019
I. S. Koh, W. Lee, *Filler Complications*, https://doi.org/10.1007/978-981-13-6639-0